the NO-NONSENSE HIV/AIDS

Shereen Usdin

'Publishers have created lists of short books that discuss the questions that your average [electoral] candidate will only ever touch if armed with a slogan and a soundbite. Together [such books] hint at a resurgence of the grand educational tradition... Closest to the hot headline issues are *The No-Nonsense Guides*. These target those topics that a large army of voters care about, but that politicos evade. Arguments, figures and documents combine to prove that good journalism is far too important to be left to (most) journalists.'

Boyd Tonkin,
The Independent,
London

The No-Nonsense Guide to HIV/AIDS
First published in the UK by
New Internationalist™ Publications Ltd
55 Rectory Road
Oxford OX4 1BW, UK
www.newint.org
New Internationalist is a registered trade mark.

In association with
Verso
6 Meard Street,
London
W1F 0EG
www.versobooks.com

Cover image: Indian children taking part in a campaign to mark World AIDS Day in New Delhi, December 1, 2002. B Mathur/Reuters.

Series editor: Troth Wells
Design by Ian Nixon / New Internationalist Publications Ltd.

Printed by TJ International Ltd, Padstow, Cornwall, UK.

British Library Cataloguing-in-Publication Data.
A catalogue record for this book is available from the British Library.

Library of Congress Cataloguing-in-Publication Data.
A catalogue for this book is available from the Library of Congress.

ISBN 1-85984-459-6

the **NO-NONSENSE** guide to
HIV/AIDS

Shereen Usdin

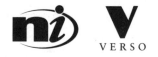
VERSO

Acknowledgements
Special thanks to Mark Heywood, Morna Cornell, Karen Usdin, Nikki Schaay, Nathan Geffen, Matthew Krouse and Mark Berger for their invaluable input. Thanks also to editor, Troth Wells for her insights and encouragement. I would also like to acknowledge all the brave people throughout the world, combating the HIV/AIDS pandemic in ways both big and small.

About the author
Shereen Usdin is a medical doctor and a public health specialist. She is co-founder of the internationally acclaimed Soul City Institute for Health and Development Communication in South Africa and works in the areas of development communication, HIV/AIDS, violence against women, health and human rights.

Other titles in the series
The No-Nonsense Guide to Globalization
The No-Nonsense Guide to Fair Trade
The No-Nonsense Guide to Climate Change
The No-Nonsense Guide to International Migration
The No-Nonsense Guide to Sexual Diversity
The No-Nonsense Guide to World History
The No-Nonsense Guide to Democracy
The No-Nonsense Guide to Class, Caste and Hierarchies
The No-Nonsense Guide to the Arms Trade
The No-Nonsense Guide to International Development
The No-Nonsense Guide to Indigenous Peoples
The No-Nonsense Guide to Terrorism
The No-Nonsense Guide to World Poverty

Foreword

It is with pleasure that I write this foreword to Shereen Usdin's thoroughly readable *No-Nonsense Guide to HIV/AIDS*. It is challenging and insightful, making a complex terrain accessible to a wide audience.

The HIV pandemic has exposed the best and worst aspects of globalization. There is tremendous hope offered by global solidarity for and by people with HIV/AIDS. Campaigns across countries such as South Africa, Kenya, Thailand, Brazil, Japan, the European Union and the United States have led to real gains for people with HIV in countries of the South.

It is also through globalization that medicines made in India or Brazil can be used in other countries such as South Africa or Botswana, or that the skills of scientists trained in the South can be used to develop life-saving medicines at US universities and vice versa. The challenge of globalization is to ensure that its benefits reach all people.

Unfortunately, however, the negative aspects of globalization have often stood in the way of progress. Inappropriate patent regimens have been forced on many countries and the strength of multinational pharmaceutical corporations has been used to intimidate countries of the South out of importing or manufacturing generic medicines. As a result, only a fraction of those who need treatment have access to life-saving medicines. Despite this unacceptable scenario, substantial progress is being made. Countries such as Brazil, where activists and government have pulled out all the stops to address the epidemic through a large-scale continuum of prevention, care and treatment, have debunked the myth that solutions to the epidemic in the South must necessarily be modest and exclude treatment.

Nevertheless, there is a growing global movement for treatment activism and its successes can be measured in increasing openness about HIV, reduced HIV medicine prices and the establishment of the Global Fund to Fight AIDS, TB and Malaria.

The lessons from the successes of solidarity over the HIV pandemic must be used in other struggles for justice if we are to build a global respect for human rights, democracy, environment and human welfare.

The history and politics of HIV, the manipulations of the pharmaceutical industry, the struggles against the disease in many parts of the world and the global solidarity of people working to alleviate this pandemic are the main themes of this book. It is an excellent guide for anyone interested in understanding the disease, the numerous forces responsible for its spread and what must be done to eradicate it.

Zackie Achmat
Chair, Treatment Action Campaign
Johannesburg

the **NO-NONSENSE** guide to

HIV/AIDS

CONTENTS

the | **NO-NONSENSE** | guide to

HIV / AIDS

The HIV/AIDS pandemic has indelibly altered the landscape of life in the 21st century. A pandemic of superlatives, it is described as the greatest humanitarian crisis the world has ever known, with millions of people either infected or affected. We are drowning in numbers. It is easy to lose perspective and become despondent.

But HIV/AIDS is also an epidemic of hope. It has given birth to social movements and community responses that reaffirm the right of life and the resilience of the human spirit. The scenario is bad but something can be done, even more so with the advent of life-prolonging medication. The grim predictions can be challenged but only if we galvanize and focus our energies and resources now.

Despite this, the world has been slow to respond. Some have argued that only once the HIV virus began to infect the heterosexual middle classes did countries in the North begin to do something about it at home, and only once it was shown to threaten global security did they begin to do something about it internationally. The jury is still out on whether governments will translate their commitments into action. With a few exceptions, countries of the South have also been slow to respond and tragically, HIV/AIDS is now reversing many of the development gains made over the last half century. To make matters worse, life-saving antiretroviral medication, which has transformed HIV/AIDS into a chronic disease in countries of the North, remains largely inaccessible to most countries of the South. This is as a result of profiteering by multinational pharmaceutical companies and the wealthy nations that protect them.

AIDS is a political issue, fuelled by poverty and gender inequalities. This *No-Nonsense Guide* examines the history and politics of the epidemic, the factors intensifying its spread and what needs to be done to turn the tide.

As a South African, my work in the field of HIV/AIDS began in the 1980s, during the last decade of the anti-apartheid struggle. South Africa's apartheid past created fertile ground for the virus to spread with large-scale social dislocation, poverty and underdevelopment. As a result, South Africa today has the highest number of people living with HIV/AIDS in the world. This brings with it a particular sadness – that millions will not be able to enjoy the fruits of our struggle for democracy. This stands to change however, if the Government keeps its recent promise to make anti-retroviral medication available to those in need. Today, HIV/AIDS is described as our 'new struggle'. Every day we witness stories of tremendous compassion and courage. And as with apartheid, with a combination of political will, mass mobilization, collective action and the necessary resources, the global HIV/AIDS pandemic can also be eradicated.

Shereen Usdin
Johannesburg

1 New world disorder

'A new world war has begun, but now it is against humanity as a whole. In the name of globalization this modern war assassinates and forgets. As in all world wars, what is at stake is a new division of the world. This new division of the world consists of increasing the power of the powerful and the misery of the miserable. The new division of the world excludes so-called minorities: indigenous peoples, youth, women, gays, lesbians, people of color, immigrants, workers, peasants. But these are actually the majority who form the global underclass – those who, in the eyes of the powerful, are dispensable. In reality this new division of the world excludes the majority.'

Subcommandante Marcos, leader of the Zapatista National Liberation Front, Mexico, 1996.

Arguably the most devastating disease ever, HIV/AIDS leaves no country untouched. Despite warnings, global responses have been slow and inadequate. Efforts have been hampered by racism, homophobia, stigma, gender inequality and deep poverty. However, doomsday predictions can be avoided if we act now. Some countries have shown that action can make all the difference.

IF SOMEONE MALICIOUS wanted to create a modern catastrophe, it would be hard to conjure up a recipe more disastrous than HIV/AIDS. These are the ingredients:

1 Take a virus that is by its nature incurable.

2 Ensure the virus can mutate, weakening the effect of drugs that help to slow down its spread, and making a vaccine elusive.

3 Spread it initially through communities already marginalized and discriminated against such as gay people, sex-workers and intravenous drug users, providing ammunition for fundamentalists looking for

'moral' scapegoats and allowing millions of vulnerable people (who may not be gay, sex-workers or intravenous drug users) to deny they are at risk.

4 Associate it directly with sex and death, creating fear and denial.

5 Let it loose on a world rife with:
- poverty and gender inequality where people have limited access to health and health services or the means to protect themselves against the circumstances in which the virus is spread.
- conflict, war and migration, resulting in great mobility and instability. In such circumstances, the incidence of rape increases or people simply seek sexual comfort where it can be found, and generally have more immediate threats to life than getting infected with HIV.

Add to this the fact that most people the world over find it difficult to talk about sex, especially to younger people, and therefore are not able to protect themselves or equip the world's youth to do so. Mix all the ingredients together to form a lethal concoction of stigma and discrimination which prevents both individuals and nations taking the necessary steps to halt the epidemic in its tracks. Allow to stew on the stove for decades through lack of political will and commitment and in very little time, the result is a major pandemic.

In just over two decades since the epidemic became visible, HIV/AIDS has spread to every corner of the world. It has infected over 60 million people, claiming almost 22 million lives. This is the equivalent of 7,000 World Trade Center 9/11 disasters, 4 Holocausts and more than 22 genocides in Rwanda. By the time you read this, it will have risen even higher.

Number-crunching around this epidemic is a depressing endeavor. At the close of the second year of the new millennium, the United Nations (UN) global estimates of people living with HIV/AIDS – shortened to 'PWAs' – stood at 42 million adults and children, most of them in sub-Saharan Africa. Five million people

Drowning by numbers

In only two decades, HIV/AIDS has mushroomed into an unprecedented global pandemic. While some countries have successfully stabilized or reversed the growing trend, the disease continues to march unchecked through most regions of the world.

Global summary of the HIV/AIDS epidemic, December 2002

Number of people living with HIV/AIDS	Total	42,000,000
	Adults	38,600,000
	Women	*19,200,000*
	Children under 15 years	3,200,000
People newly infected with HIV in 2002	Total	5,000,000
	Adults	4,200,000
	Women	*2,000,000*
	Children under 15 years	800,000
AIDS deaths in 2002	Total	3,100,000
	Adults	2,500,000
	Women	*1,200,000*
	Children under 15 years	610,000

AIDS Epidemic Update, UNAIDS, December 2002. www.unaids.org

were infected in the year 2002 alone. In the same year, 3 million people died of AIDS; by 2002 14 million children were orphaned.[1,2] According to UNAIDS, HIV/AIDS is now by far the leading cause of death in sub-Saharan Africa, and the fourth biggest global killer. It is impacting on the world in both the private and the public spheres of life at all levels, yet HIV is elusive to track. Stigma leads people to hide the disease – 'he died of tuberculosis (TB), not AIDS' is a typical response. Predictions, based as they are on different theoretical models and assumptions, are also subject to lively debate. While some contest the accuracy of the UN figures, no-one doubts the huge impact of AIDS, threatening every aspect of development and setting back the gains made over the last five decades.

The epidemic's effect on life expectancy is alarming. In a world without AIDS, the average citizen of sub-Saharan Africa could expect to live for 62 years. With AIDS, she or he will be lucky to reach a 47th birthday. Life expectancy in Botswana has dropped to 39 years, compared with the prediction of 72 years without AIDS – taking the country back to levels of over 50 years ago. The especially deep impact of the disease in Africa south of the Sahara gives this book a strong focus on that region.

From the early 1980s, when AIDS was a footnote in most medical textbooks, it has spawned a generation of scientists, development workers, activists and academics. From a marginalized disease of 'gay men in San Francisco' or Africans, which a largely homophobic and racist world ignored, the epidemic is now a concern of the international community, discussed at the highest level in both the North and South. It is probably the most researched medical and social problem in the world, the stuff of international conferences attracting thousands of people. It is finally – after years of inaction – on the agenda of global summits and decision-making forums – from the G8 (the world's richest countries plus Russia) to the World Economic Forum, and more recently even the UN Security Council – the first time the Council has ever debated a health or development issue. Still, political commitment from the 'First World' to address the pandemic remains inadequate.

Far-reaching effects

While figures are thrown around, AIDS' far-reaching effects can never be fully told in numbers. For every one person infected, countless others are affected directly or indirectly. The resounding slogan of AIDS in the new millennium is 'we are *all* infected or affected'.

Like other major calamities, AIDS has brought out both the best and the worst in us. On the one hand, it has taken some back to darker ages, where the fear of the unknown or the incurable has resulted in acts of enormous cruelty. On the other hand, many people have accomplished extraordinary things – mobilizing emotional, financial and other resources to take care of community members and loved ones who are HIV-positive. Stories of astounding courage and generosity of spirit have emerged. And in a world where money can still buy you life, activists – like David against Goliath – have taken on powerful transnational drug companies and governments to fight for access to lifesaving drugs.

When did it all start?

Nobody knows exactly when HIV made its first appearance but scientists have found traces of HIV in the blood of a man who died in the Congo (now DR Congo) in 1959. A Manchester sailor is thought to have died of an AIDS-like illness in the same year but this remains unconfirmed. Scientists speculate – based on the time it takes for genetic changes to occur – that the virus must have been around for many years before this.

The early 1980s were turbulent years on many fronts – the Cold War wrought global havoc and space exploration reached new heights. It was also during these years that HIV first became visible. However, the current epidemic probably started in the mid to late 1970s when several cases of what would later be called AIDS were reported in the US, Sweden, Tanzania and Haiti.

Why did it all start? Monkeys or the CIA?

While the exact origins of HIV are not known, it is generally accepted that the virus crossed over from a species of monkey in Africa in the early 1900s. HIV-1, one of the two major strains of HIV, is thought to have spread from chimpanzees to humans in central Africa. In West Africa, the less aggressive HIV-2 strain is believed to have spread from macaque monkeys.[3] The spread of viruses across species is not a rare phenomenon. It happens with various strains of flu where viruses are passed on through an animal host or reservoir, to humans. The conclusion that this is the origin of AIDS is based on the similarities between the human and monkey forms of the virus as well the common geography shared by both the monkeys' and the human viral strains. While the definitive answer as to

A global snapshot

By the end of 2002, no part of the world was unaffected. Low prevalence rates in highly populated regions such as Asia and the Pacific can be deceptive. In India for example, an estimated prevalence rate of less than 1 per cent amounts to almost 4 million people, making it second only to South Africa in terms of sheer numbers of people living with HIV.

Regional HIV/AIDS statistics and features, end of 2002

Region	Epidemic started	Adults and children living with HIV/AIDS	Adults and children newly infected with HIV	Adult prevalence rate*	% of HIV-positive adults who are women	Main mode(s) of transmission# for adults living with HIV/AIDS
Sub-Saharan Africa	late 70s, early 80s	29,400,000	3,500,000	8.8%	58%	Hetero
North Africa & Middle East	late 80s	550,000	83,000	0.3%	55%	Hetero, IDU
South & South-East Asia	late 80s	6,000,000	700,000	0.6%	36%	Hetero, DU
East Asia & Pacific	late 80s	1,200,000	270,000	0.1%	24%	IDU, hetero, MSM
Latin America	late 70s, early 80s	1,500,000	150,000	0.6%	30%	MSM, IDU, hetero
Caribbean	late 70s, early 80s	440,000	60,000	2.4%	50%	Hetero, MSM
Eastern Europe & Central Asia	early 90s	1,200,000	250,000	0.6%	27%	IDU
Western Europe	late 70s, early 80s	570,000	30,000	0.3%	25%	MSM, IDU
North America	late 70s, early 80s	980,000	45,000	0.6%	20%	MSM, IDU, hetero
Australia & NZ	late 70s, early 80s	15,000	500	0.1%	7%	MSM
TOTAL		**42,000,000**	**5,000,000**	**1.2%**	**50%**	

* The proportion of adults (15 to 49 years of age) living with HIV/AIDS in 2002, using 2002 population numbers.
\# Hetero (heterosexual transmission), IDU (transmission through injecting drug use), MSM (sexual transmission among men who have sex with men).

AIDS Epidemic Update, UNAIDS, December 2002. www.unaids.org

how this happened is anyone's guess, there has been much speculation. Perhaps the most likely scenario is that the virus spread to humans around the 1930s as a result of blood from an infected monkey contaminating a cut on the hand of a hunter or person preparing the monkey meat for cooking.[4] Some scientists believe the virus may well have crossed the species barrier even earlier and petered out. During the 1930s however, the virus found fertile ground for rapid global spread because of the human traffic during the colonial and post-colonial periods in Africa along with the development of modern transport infrastructure.[5]

Polio vaccine

Another theory is that the virus may have crossed over from monkeys to humans as a result of incubating polio vaccines in chimpanzee kidneys. Some argue that the virus was then inoculated into people during the 1950s' polio vaccination campaigns in central Africa. In 2000 a phial of polio vaccine that was used in this campaign was discovered in the stores of the Wistar Institute in Philadelphia. It was tested but no trace of HIV was found.[6]

A rather dubious line of argument is that the virus was actually created in a laboratory as a form of biological warfare. This highly unlikely proposition has been espoused by a few prominent leaders including Sam Nujoma, President of Namibia, who is on record as saying: 'It is also an historical fact that HIV/AIDS is a man-made disease, it is not natural.' At the 2001 African AIDS Summit in Nigeria, Colonel Muammar Qadhafi, President of Libya, took this to its conspiratorial extreme: 'Who created the AIDS virus?' he asked. 'It is the laboratories of the CIA. They played around with viruses until they managed to create this one.'[7] Notorious Ku Klux Klan supporter William Cooper claims that AIDS has been deliberately manufactured by the Illuminati (allegedly a secret society of the world's most powerful) to rid the world of homosexuals and certain racial groups.[8] While many Africans humorously interpret the AIDS acronym as 'American Invention to Discourage Sex [in Africa]' the idea of the sinister and intentional use of HIV for political gain is not entirely unfounded. The infamous South African scientist, Dr Wouter Basson, also known as 'Dr Death', was employed by the apartheid regime in the 1980s to devise ways to eliminate its opponents. Father of South Africa's first biological warfare program, he has also been accused of sending out HIV-positive spies to deliberately infect the black population.

In truth, the origins of AIDS would be irrelevant if it weren't important to understand how the virus mutates and progresses over time. This helps doctors predict where the epidemic is headed and provides vital information for scientists developing vaccines and treatments. The problem however with dwelling on the epidemic's roots is that people distort the speculations to apportion blame and to create scapegoats, feeding into racism and xenophobia. A journalist once asked DR Congo's top AIDS specialist whether the reason AIDS was such a problem in Africa was because people were having sex with monkeys.[9]

First signs

Most people wouldn't look to epidemiology – the study of disease patterns – for a thrilling career. And yet the discovery of the HIV virus reads like a detective novel and has even become the stuff of feature films.

In March 1981, doctors in the US began to notice a strange phenomenon. Kaposi's Sarcoma (KS) – a relatively rare form of cancer – started to appear in an aggressive form in about eight young gay men in New York. It startled doctors because they were used to seeing the disease mainly in elderly men. Around this time Sandra Ford, a drug technician at the US Centers for Disease Control (CDC) in Atlanta, was perturbed by the sudden increase in requests for the drug Pentamine, used for the treatment of a rare lung infection called pneumocystis carinii pneumonia (PCP). In an interview with *Newsweek* she described her concerns: 'A doctor was treating a gay man in his twenties who had pneumonia. Two weeks later, he called to ask for a refill of a rare drug that I handled. This was unusual – nobody ever asked for a refill. Patients usually were cured in one 10-day-treatment or they died.'[10] PCP was also turning up in a small group of men in Los Angeles and New York.

In June 1981, the CDC set up a task force on KS and 'opportunistic infections' (diseases like tuberculosis [TB] that strike a weakened immune system) to track the problem and determine the cause of this unusual situation. At this stage, having appeared only among gay men, the disease was not thought to be contagious. It was even described medically as 'gay compromise syndrome' or 'GRID' (gay-related immune deficiency). A few months later however, PCP was detected in inject-ing drug users. In our homophobic and intolerant world, these first 'sightings' of HIV in already margin-alized communities laid the foundation for much of the stigma we see today. By August 1982, the disease finally got a name: AIDS – an acronym for Acquired Immune Deficiency Syndrome (SIDA in Spanish and French). Soon cases started cropping up all over America, with reports of HIV also in Haiti and Britain.

It was only around 1982, when AIDS was identified in hemophiliac patients who had received blood trans-fusions that fears began to emerge that AIDS could be the result of something infectious. News spread fast and public hysteria followed. Police wore special masks and gloves when dealing with 'suspected AIDS patients'. 'Suspects' ranged from protesters at gay ral-lies to accident victims.[11] The term 'gay plague' or 'gay cancer' was coined by the media.

Slims disease

Around this time scientists in Uganda were also start-ing to put two and two together. In 1983 David

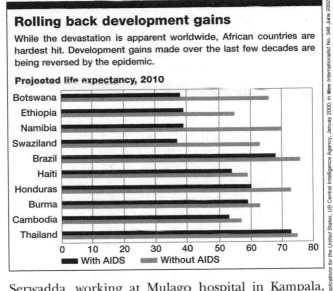

Rolling back development gains

While the devastation is apparent worldwide, African countries are hardest hit. Development gains made over the last few decades are being reversed by the epidemic.

Projected life expectancy, 2010

Botswana
Ethiopia
Namibia
Swaziland
Brazil
Haiti
Honduras
Burma
Cambodia
Thailand

0   10   20   30   40   50   60   70   80

■ With AIDS   ▧ Without AIDS

The Global Infectious Disease Threat and its implications for the United States, US Central Intelligence Agency, January 2000, in *New Internationalist* No. 346 June 2002.

Serwadda, working at Mulago hospital in Kampala, began to notice male and female patients with KS – all from the Rakai district of the country. With KS only common in elderly Ugandan men, Serwadda was alarmed. He and other local doctors were also becoming increasingly frustrated because their Rakai patients with TB or malaria were not improving on treatment. On the contrary, they seemed to be getting worse or responding momentarily, only to contract new infections. Serwadda began corresponding with Anne Bayley, a cancer surgeon in Zambia. Bayley was seeing a similar phenomenon with KS in patients suffering from what became known in Africa as Slims disease, because of the wasted appearance of those affected. Bayley suspected a connection between Slims disease and AIDS. This was confirmed a few years later when Serwadda sent off blood samples from some of his patients to London for testing: all came back positive for HIV.[12] In 1983 medical science reported that the disease could be passed on heterosexually.

The race to make history

The human immunodeficiency virus was first isolated in May 1983 by Luc Montagnier at the French Institut Pasteur. Researchers called it LAV (lymphadenopathy-associated virus) and suspected it was the cause of AIDS but little attention was paid until the following year, when the French announced further research that confirmed this finding. In a flurry of activity, the US Government suddenly declared that Dr Robert Gallo of the National Cancer Institute had discovered the virus that caused AIDS. They called the virus HTLV-3 (human T-cell lymphotrophic virus, type 3) and predicted that a vaccine would be available within two years. Almost 20 years later, a vaccine remains elusive. It took some time before everyone realized that LAV and HTLV-3 were the same thing and in 1986, both names were replaced by Human Immunodeficiency Virus (HIV). In the interim, however, a nasty spat between the US and France had ensued, each claiming to be the first to discover the virus. Making big money as well as big history were both at stake and in 1985, following the race to develop and patent the first HIV test, the French Institut sued the National Cancer Institute for a share of the royalties of the patented test. France ultimately won the 'accolade' and was officially declared to have discovered HIV. More recently, Montagnier and Gallo have joined forces to develop a vaccine for HIV.

But in the meantime, the world remained baffled as to how the virus was spreading from one person to another. Fears of casual transmission abounded when AIDS was first reported in children. In 1983, for the first time, the concept of mother-to-child transmission (MTCT) appeared on the radar screen. By around 1986, AIDS had cropped up in every region of the globe and the world was hungry for a scapegoat. Stigma and discrimination were already setting in, providing a field day for rampant homophobia and xenophobia as first gay people and later Africans bore the brunt. Stories emerged of people evicted from their homes, fired from their jobs and ostracized by their communities upon revealing that they were HIV-positive.

In 1985, Ryan White, a young American with hemophilia, was banned from school when people learned he was HIV-positive. Gradually, however, despite their fear of anyone and everyone with HIV, people began to divide the world into those who were perceived to be 'innocent victims' of HIV – children and hemophiliacs – and those who were 'guilty'– like gay men, sex-workers and injecting drug users: people seen as 'getting their just desserts'.

Activism under way

While the gay community in the US was being stigmatized, it was also at the forefront of the response to the epidemic, forming organizations to educate the public, support the sick and dying and to protect people's rights. In 1986, the AIDS Coalition To Unleash Power (ACT UP) was founded to fight the lack of a political response to AIDS. According to Eric Sawyer of the organization's New York chapter: 'Activism happened in the US primarily because we were fighting for our lives. We responded as a community fighting a war. We took to the streets; we took care of our brothers and our sisters in our homes. We really joined together with a sense of a community, to respond as if we were under attack by a foreign military.'[13]

It was the activism of the gay community that forced the US Government out of its initial denial. In 1981, the year Ronald Reagan was sworn in as President, 422 cases of AIDS had been diagnosed in the US and 159 people were dead. By 1986, over 42,000 cases of AIDS had been diagnosed there and close on 25,000 people were dead. Despite this, Reagan only mentioned the word AIDS for the first time in public in 1987, six years after the epidemic 'began'.[14] Even then he got it horribly wrong, calling for the AIDS virus to be added to the list of contagious diseases for which 'immigrants and aliens seeking permanent residence in the US can be denied entry'. The US Government like most other governments in this context was criminally slow to react. Many argue that it was only once heterosexual America began to feel threatened that anything substantial happened. Compare this for example to the US's rapid response to Legionnaire's Disease which broke out in 1976 among small numbers of middle-class heterosexuals in Philadelphia.

Reframing the epidemic

It was fast becoming clear that AIDS – perceived initially as a medical problem – was actually a social problem requiring a broader response. In October 1987 AIDS became the first disease ever debated on the floor of the UN General Assembly. The Global Program on AIDS (GPA) was formed under the auspices of the World Health Organization (WHO) with the promise to mobilize the entire UN system in the worldwide struggle against AIDS. The GPA catalyzed resources and galvanized action. Petty politics in WHO intervened however, and GPA head Jonathan Mann was effectively forced to resign. The GPA was disbanded but not before Mann and his team had successfully reframed HIV and AIDS as a social problem and highlighted for the first time the human rights dimensions of the epidemic (see chapter 5).

Civil society organizations around the world were at the forefront of the struggle, saying 'enough was enough' and calling for an end to silence, discrimination and inaction.

Scare tactics

Regrettably, scare tactics were the order of the day in the initial campaigns designed to alert the public to the dangers of AIDS. The effect was to exacerbate discrimination and stigma. In 1987, the Australian Government launched a campaign showing AIDS as the 'Grim Reaper' – a rotting corpse with a scythe –

playing a lethal game of death in a bowling alley. Mowing down pins of real people, the message was clear – AIDS KILLS. In South Africa, the first awareness campaigns focused on funerals and hopelessness. British public service adverts on TV showed volcanoes erupting to music reminiscent of the soundtrack to the movie 'Jaws'.

Despite the shock value, nobody seemed to change behavior as a result and many newly diagnosed people, fearful that death was imminent, committed suicide or closed their businesses, sold their assets and prepared for the worst. Educators began to realize that these campaigns were only heightening fear and hysteria and so shifted the focus to convey the notion that HIV was not a death sentence. People could live for many healthy and productive years with HIV before becoming sick with AIDS, and even then adopting a healthy lifestyle with good nutrition and aggressive treatment of opportunistic infections like TB and thrush were prolonging life further. Insulting and misleading terms such as 'sufferers or victims' were replaced with more politically and descriptively correct terms such as People Living With HIV/AIDS (PWAs). While stigma fomented the silence around AIDS a few role models began to speak out. Celebrity basketball star Magic Johnson and tennis ace Arthur Ashe revealed that they were HIV-positive. Princess Diana openly hugged people with AIDS. Zambia's President Kaunda told the world that his son was HIV-positive.

'Lazarus effect'

In 1987 AZT, the world's first antiretroviral (ARV) drug was finally approved by the US Food and Drug Administration (FDA) for use by PWAs in the US. The FDA had dragged its feet for years on this issue until public protest, particularly ACT UP's confrontational civil disobedience campaigns, forced its hand. Living positively with HIV/AIDS became even more of a possibility with ARVs which – although not a cure – slow down the replication of the virus, thereby extending both the quality and the length of life. ACT UP protested for over two more years before successfully pressuring Burroughs Wellcome, manufacturer of AZT, to lower its exorbitant price in North America by 20 per cent. Even then, it remained out of reach for most people with HIV in the world.

In 1995 a major drug trial showed that combinations of two ARVs were better than one and a year later, triple therapy became the standard treatment of choice. In what became referred to as the 'Lazarus effect', people at death's door literally came back to life. These drugs began to change the course of the epidemic in wealthier countries, from a fatal illness to a chronic disease not unlike diabetes or hypertension. In 1996 Magic Johnson, by now on antiretroviral medication, announced his return to professional basketball.

Also by 1996, savvy prevention campaigns and the advent of drugs began to turn the tide of the epidemic in some parts of the world with UNAIDS reporting a slowing down in the North and in parts of Africa. Marking a turning point, the first AIDS hospice in San Francisco closed as fewer people were dying of the disease.[15] Uganda, after a decade of denial, was also beginning to show success with figures of HIV in pregnant women in Kampala dropping from around 30 to 11 per cent between 1992 and 2000.[16] By 2002, the use of ARVs together with breastmilk substitutes had virtually eliminated the pediatric AIDS epidemic in countries of the North.

Widening inequalities

Precious time passed however, and the virus tightened its hold in Africa, especially south of the Sahara. Households sank deeper into poverty as economically active family members became sick or died and other income earners in the family stayed home to care for them. Families sold their meager assets to pay for

> '*Let us not equivocate. AIDS today in Africa is claiming more lives than the sum total of all wars, famines and floods, and the ravages of such deadly diseases as malaria. It is devastating families and communities.*' ∎
>
> Nelson Mandela, former President of South Africa.

healthcare and funerals. A generation of teachers, health-workers, police and civil servants has been placed in jeopardy, undermining the provision of social services and potentially resulting in serious social instability. Many years will pass before the private sector wakes up to the significant effect the epidemic will have on their bottom line as their employees become sick and die (see chapter 2). The impact on children has been an unfolding tragedy with consequences for generations to come. Children, usually girls, have been forced to leave school to look after their sick parents. Africa began to report the rising phenomenon of 'child-headed households' as young children fended for themselves when their parents died. While many families, often already destitute, opened their homes to these children, large numbers remain homeless and vulnerable to exploitation and abuse. Clearly, many people rose to the epidemic's challenge and continue to do so today. Community initiatives sprang up all over the continent to educate and to support PWAs. Home-based care for those in need has become widespread.

At this stage, it was becoming obvious to many that AIDS was deepening the existing inequality between the North and South. While profits from expensive ARVs were lining the pockets of shareholders in multinational drug companies and addressing the epidemic for the rich, the South was left to mobilize care and support for the sick and the dying. Projects were orientated towards helping PWAs to 'die with dignity'. An outraged Major Rubaramira Ruranga from Uganda who pioneered much of the country's AIDS prevention program in the military railed against this injustice:

'What is dying with dignity? Why do you train me to die with dignity when actually I should not die?'[17]

But by the mid-1990s the injustice was glaring and AIDS activists throughout the world began to ask the obvious question: 'What about drugs for the South?' At the 1996 international AIDS Conference, Noerine Kalleba of UNAIDS in Uganda said: 'We have heard… about the exciting advances that have been made with regard to the use of AZT in interrupting mother-to-child transmission of HIV. The young infected woman in Africa is asking where, how, when does she access this?'[18] Seven years later Kalleba would still be asking this question.

In the 1990s, the site of struggle shifted to get the global community to wake up to the devastating impact of HIV in the South. Yet the world continued to react with an astounding lack of urgency. In 1995, a

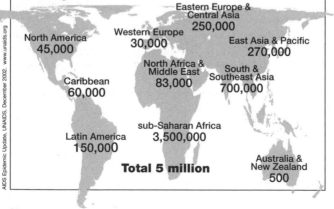

The rising tide

While the vast majority of existing and new infections are located in sub-Saharan Africa, the epidemic is growing most rapidly in regions such as Eastern Europe and Asia. In Asia and the Pacific regions, the number of people living with HIV/AIDS increased by 10 per cent between 2001 and 2002.

Estimated number of adults and children newly infected with HIV during 2002

Eastern Europe & Central Asia
250,000

North America
45,000

Western Europe
30,000

East Asia & Pacific
270,000

North Africa & Middle East
83,000

South & Southeast Asia
700,000

Caribbean
60,000

sub-Saharan Africa
3,500,000

Latin America
150,000

Total 5 million

Australia & New Zealand
500

AIDS Epidemic Update, UNAIDS, December 2002. www.unaids.org

few years after the closure of the GPA, UNAIDS was formed to bring together all UN agencies in an expanded global response. According to its head, Peter Piot, the formation was a bit half-hearted and took place in a hostile environment. Instead of increasing their spending, Piot maintained that the opposite occurred.[19]

Global response

It is fair to say that the global response to the epidemic in Africa was a reflection of racism; but also of vested interests, or lack of them. In 1990 a CIA report predicted 45 million people, the majority of them Africans, would be infected by the end of the first millennium. Walter Barrows, CIA Intelligence Analyst, admitted: 'Had the studies predicted that the bulk of the impact of the pandemic was in some other region of the world, perhaps Europe or even Asia, say Japan, probably the US policy response, probably the world response, would have been different.'[20]

A later report by the CIA advised that the increasing number of infectious diseases, especially AIDS, would pose both health and broader threats to the US and its interests. It suggested that the epidemic could negatively impact on the social, economic and political stability of countries and regions of significance to the US.[21] At last, the top US policy dogs paid attention and in 2000 the UN Security Council actually discussed AIDS as a security issue. Stephen Lewis, UN Special Envoy for HIV/AIDS in Africa, noted in response: 'No one diminishes the question of security... but it does say something about the way we respond to the human condition, doesn't it? It's not enough to engage the world simply by having an incomparable human catastrophe; it has to have security implications to make it come alive.'

Meanwhile African leaders had not responded with much alacrity either. Racist perceptions about AIDS in Africa were in some part responsible for this inaction, feeding into a pattern of AIDS denial across the continent. For example, as far into the epidemic as the late 1990s, President Mbeki of South Africa appointed a panel of scientists to determine, amongst other things, whether HIV does indeed cause AIDS – an absurd debate given the overwhelming body of evidence verifying this fact (see chapter 3). There were however, a few notable exceptions. As seen earlier, Zambia's President Kaunda went public about his son's HIV-positive status in 1987 and Uganda, after its initial period of denial, took the bull by the horns with large-scale prevention campaigns that broke taboos on talking openly about sex and instituted sexuality education for young children in schools.

The right to live

Social movements began to form in both the North and South to press for treatment access. These organizations have helped to put the issue on both their countries' and the international agenda. Access to AIDS drugs took center stage as one of the most profound ethical issues faced by the world at the end of the last century. In 2001 only 30,000 of the over 28 million infected people in sub-Saharan Africa were on treatment and over 2 million died of AIDS.[22]

In the same year, the Global Fund to Fight HIV/AIDS, TB and Malaria was established to try to assist countries to address the epidemic, in part by improving access to medication. It is estimated that the South needs US$7-10 billion a year to meet this goal. Compare this to the $300 billion rich countries spend annually on agricultural subsidies to protect their markets. Yet one year after its establishment, the Global Fund remains hopelessly under-resourced. At the time of the writing, fewer than 5 per cent of people in the South needing treatment were receiving it.

President Bush recently announced the US would give $15 billion, independent of the Global Fund, to fight the pandemic in Africa and Asia. Some of this

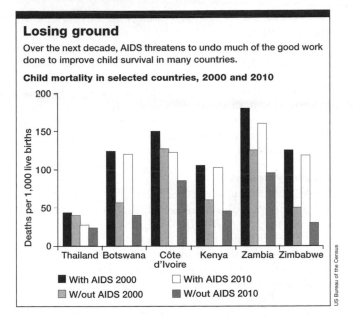

Losing ground

Over the next decade, AIDS threatens to undo much of the good work done to improve child survival in many countries.

Child mortality in selected countries, 2000 and 2010

Deaths per 1,000 live births

Thailand, Botswana, Côte d'Ivoire, Kenya, Zambia, Zimbabwe

- ■ With AIDS 2000
- □ With AIDS 2010
- ▨ W/out AIDS 2000
- ▨ W/out AIDS 2010

US Bureau of the Census

money would be available for treatment. Initially the so-called 'Gag Rule' applied – the infamous Mexico City Policy – which prevents US funding from going to any organization promoting the termination of pregnancies or providing any form of counseling, referrals, services or lobbying around abortion rights. This is an untenable condition to apply, particularly in the context of HIV/AIDS which is so tightly linked to the issue of women's reproductive rights and where termina tion is one of the choices offered to HIV-positive pregnant women.

Public outrage reversed the 'Gag Rule' but concerns remain that alternate ways of applying it will be sought through country bilaterals outside the jurisdiction of the Global Fund and also, very importantly, that the $15 billion promised will not actually be forthcoming. While activists have cautiously welcomed the money, it is viewed as inadequate, spread as it will be over 5 years and compared to the $75 billion the US spent on bombing Iraq.

What will happen if we maintain the status quo? The epidemic, which unbelievably is still in its early stages, will mushroom exponentially. Although initial predictions were that it would saturate in the worst-hit countries, it is showing no signs of letting up. There are also indications of resurgence in some countries where it was previously under control, giving no room for complacency.

Untimely deaths

UNAIDS estimates that between 2000 and 2020, 68 million people will die earlier than they would have in the absence of AIDS. In sub-Saharan Africa, where over 29 million people are infected with the virus, the predictions are that 55 million additional deaths will occur in the next 20 years. Heavily affected countries could lose more than 20 per cent of their Gross Domestic Product by 2020. According to the Food and Agricultural Organization (FAO) 7 million farm-workers worldwide have died from AIDS-related causes since 1985 and 16 million more are expected to die in the next 20 years, exacerbating already widespread food shortages. UNAIDS estimates that there will be 40 million children who will have lost their parents to AIDS.

The enormous social toll is difficult to quantify. Companies will incur increasing costs due to absenteeism and illness, insurance and benefit payouts, the death of large numbers of their workforce and the costs of training new employees. Patients with AIDS-related illnesses already occupy almost two-thirds of hospital beds in many African countries and the epidemic threatens to wreck already compromised health infrastructures.

The New Partnership for Africa's Development (NEPAD), Africa's blueprint for economic rejuvenation, aims for an annual growth rate of 7 per cent over

15 years, cutting poverty in half by the year 2015. The UN's Stephen Lewis comments: 'There will be no continuous 7 per cent annual growth rate in the 25 countries where the prevalence rate of HIV is above 5 per cent – considered to be the dangerous take-off point for the pandemic – unless the pandemic is defeated. In fact, it is virtually certain that several of those countries will experience a negative rate of growth year over year under present circumstances.'[23]

NEPAD itself acknowledges that unless communicable diseases, most particularly HIV/AIDS, are brought under control, 'real gains in human development will remain an impossible hope'.

According to the UNAIDS 2002 Report, Eastern Europe and Central Asia are now experiencing the fastest-growing epidemic in the world. However, while countries like India, China and Indonesia have low prevalence rates, because of their enormous populations they have huge numbers of HIV-positive people.

Political will moves mountains

Action can change things. The epidemic has begun to recede in countries with the political will to take strong action. Brazil, Australia, Thailand, Cambodia, Uganda and the Philippines are some of the countries where concerted efforts have reaped rewards. Early implementation of large-scale prevention and treatment programs have helped contain potentially explosive epidemics. In June 2001, the UN General Assembly brought out the Declaration of Commitment on HIV/AIDS, setting time-bound targets which member countries have committed to and to which they will be held accountable. Many nations have developed national strategies and established special councils to deal with HIV/AIDS. In 1998 UNAIDS and the Office of the UN High Commissioner for Human Rights brought out its International Guidelines on HIV/AIDS and Human Rights* and in 2002 amended one of the guidelines to recognize antiretroviral treatment as an essential component of a comprehensive response to the epidemic and fundamental to the realization of the right to health. It calls on governments to establish concrete national plans on HIV/AIDS-related treatment, with resources and timelines that progressively lead to equal and universal access to HIV/AIDS treatment, care and support. ∎

*www.unaids.org

India for example has an adult HIV prevalence rate of less than 1 per cent, but this amounts to almost 4 million people. Nigeria, Ethiopia, Russia, India and China, referred to as the 'new wave countries', are all on the cusp of major epidemics and according to UNAIDS Asia is likely to eclipse sub-Saharan Africa in absolute numbers of people living with HIV/AIDS by 2010. At this point in time, not a single country is unaffected.

While it is true that the world is starting to wake up to the enormity of HIV/AIDS, much more must be done to halt the march of the disease. The world is watching to see if countries abide by their paper promises. Graça Machel, the tireless Mozambican campaigner for human rights, made this statement at the 2002 Barcelona 14th International Conference on AIDS: 'When HIV and AIDS attack, nothing is left as it was before – for individuals, families, communities and nations. Yet our response has been appallingly weak. Unlike the virus, we have not been aggressive enough. Unlike the virus, we have not been integrated and comprehensive in our strategies. Unlike the virus, we have not been unrelenting in our commitment.'

Twenty years have passed since the HIV virus first became visible. How many more years and conferences will take place before we commit the necessary resources to turn this pandemic around?

1 Cited in *Unsustainability: a handbook for journalists* (SANGOCO, Johannesburg 2002). **2** Defined as children aged 0-14, who have lost one or both parents to AIDS. **3** T Barnett, A Whiteside, *AIDS in the Twenty-First Century: Disease and Globalization* (Palgrave Macmillan 2002) p 36. **4** T Barnett, A Whiteside, op. cit. p 37. **5** T Barnett, A Whiteside, op. cit. **6** P Blanco et al, *Nature*, 410, 1045-1046, 2001. Cited on www.avert.org/origins.htm **7** P Brooks 'An Account of a Catastrophe Foretold', *Steps for the Future* television series, 2001. **8** W Cooper, *Behold a Pale Horse* (Light Technology Publishing: Flagstaff, Arizona, USA, 1991). **9** Interview with Peter Piot in P Brooks, 'An Account of a Catastrophe Foretold', *Steps for the Future* television series, 2001. **10** D McGinn, 'MSNBC: AIDS at 20: Anatomy of a Plague; an Oral History', *Newsweek Web Exclusive* (http://www.msnbc.com/news/581827.asp) cited on www.avert.org/his81_86.htm **11** A Kanabus, J Fredriksson, *A History of AIDS*. www.avert.org/his81-86.htm (26 June 2002). **12** H Marais, S Usdin, M Cornell, 'The Deadly Denial of Africa's Baptism of AIDS', *Sunday Independent* (South Africa), 22 October 2000. **13** P Brooks, 'An Account of a Catastrophe Foretold', *Steps for the Future* television series. **14** A Kanabus and J Fredriksson, 'A History of AIDS', *AVERT,* www.avert.org/his81-86.htm. **15** www.avert.org/his93_97.htm **16** 'Report on the Global HIV/AIDS Epidemic', *UNAIDS Report, 2002.* **17** P Brooks, 'An Account of a Catastrophe Foretold', *Steps for the Future* television series, 2001. **18** P Brooks, op. cit. **19** P Brooks, op.cit. **20** P Brooks, op. cit. **21** David Gordon, CIA analyst interviewed in: P Brooks, op. cit. **22** *Business Day* (South Africa), 3 July 2002. **23** S Lewis speech on G7, NEPAD, cited on AF-AIDS 2002.

2 'Why us, why now?' – what is fuelling the epidemic

'The microbe is nothing; the terrain, everything.'
Louis Pasteur, 19th century French scientist.[1]

While AIDS is seen by many as a plague to punish 21st century Earth, the fact is that it is caused by the Human Immunodeficiency Virus (HIV) and, like all diseases, has a biological explanation. It does not discriminate or target particular groups for 'punishment'. Anyone is vulnerable if placed at risk, but there are factors that make some people more vulnerable – such as being a woman or being poor – and create ideal conditions for the virus to spread.

SOUTH AFRICA'S PRESIDENT Thabo Mbeki incurred the wrath of AIDS workers throughout the world by implying that poverty is the cause of AIDS. The President did not help matters with his musings on whether or not a virus was responsible in any way for the epidemic. Of course, poverty cannot *cause* AIDS – the Human Immunodeficiency Virus must be present. However there is no doubt that, as with many other diseases, poverty creates a social and economic environment that encourages the spread of the virus. While wealthier people are not immune, the epidemic clearly follows the fault lines of poverty and social upheaval.

Despite the deluge of media images of carefree people living it up in luxurious holiday destinations, 21st century Earth is not a pretty place. The combined income of the 582 million people living in the 43 least developed countries is $146 billion compared to the $1 trillion combined wealth of the world's 200 richest people. After years of colonialism, wars, poor governance, debt and structural adjustment, many countries are spiraling into crises, resulting in hotbeds for epidemics like AIDS, TB and malaria to spread.

Josephine Mangodza in Zimbabwe describes an all-too-common reality (see box).

(i) HIV/AIDS and poverty

The first part of this chapter looks in more detail at how poverty affects the epidemic and vice versa. Around 6 billion people inhabit our world. Of these, more than 1 million live on less than $1 a day and do not have access to the most basic necessities of life – food, water, sanitation, housing, health care and education. One-sixth of the world's people are malnourished.

In a recent study of countries in southern Africa, people were asked how often their family has gone without enough food to eat in the last 12 months. Of the respondents, 80 per cent in Lesotho said 'sometimes' or 'often'; in Namibia, it was 71 per cent; 77 per cent in Zimbabwe; 69 per cent in Zambia and Malawi.

This is a horrible reality but what does it have to do with AIDS? Unfortunately, the links are inextricable. According to UNAIDS and WHO, most of the 42 million people currently infected with HIV live in poor countries in the developing world, with 29 million of these in sub-Saharan Africa. Of the 40 'least developed' members of the United Nations, 32 are located in this region.[2] The implications are sobering – poverty renders populations more vulnerable to HIV/AIDS and the epidemic then deepens poverty. While Africa is worst affected, economic crises are also driving the spread of the disease elsewhere. UNAIDS' 2000 Report notes that mass unemployment and poverty together with deteriorating public health and social services are behind the growing epidemic in Eastern Europe.

While AIDS is busy undoing the development gains of recent times – contested, uneven or meager as those gains may be – the epidemic is also lodging among poorer populations in high-income countries. Despite its decline amongst better-off whites in the US, infection rates are rising amongst poorer black and Hispanic populations there. A similar pattern is emerging in Canada where rates amongst indigenous populations increased by 90 per cent from 1997 to 1999.

Poverty's effects

How exactly does poverty fuel the epidemic? Simply put, being poor reduces people's options in life. For example, faced with the prospect of starvation now or illness later, millions of people (women in particular) are forced into sex work to keep their families alive.

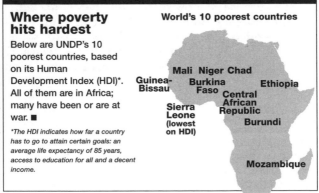

Where poverty hits hardest

World's 10 poorest countries

Below are UNDP's 10 poorest countries, based on its Human Development Index (HDI)*. All of them are in Africa; many have been or are at war. ■

*The HDI indicates how far a country has to go to attain certain goals: an average life expectancy of 85 years, access to education for all and a decent income.

Guinea-Bissau Mali Niger Chad Burkina Faso Central African Republic Ethiopia Sierra Leone (lowest on HDI) Burundi Mozambique

Source: Human Development Report, UNDP 2001.

Denise, a Namibian sex-worker, had to make this difficult choice in order to put bread on her table: 'I am not happy with what I do but I have to do it because I must survive. I must keep my children alive. Some days there is not even bread at home; then I have to go out and earn money. My father was a fisherman until last year when he got a stroke and was laid off. My husband died last year. I know it [sex work] is illegal in Namibia but I have no choice; there is no other income.'[3]

The virus has taken hold among India's poorest people where the first AIDS cases were detected amongst destitute women struggling to support their families through sex work. Fifty per cent of the country's blood supply comes from poor people selling their blood to survive and initially many cases of HIV transmission there occurred through transfusions with unscreened infected blood. This has also been the case in China where the majority of the country's 3 million paid donors come from impoverished rural communities. Lack of basic blood donation safety procedures resulted in wide-scale infections, with subsequent spread through sexual contact.[4]

Poverty and unemployment also increase relationships of dependency making women more vulnerable to coercive and risky sex. Try negotiating 'safer sex' with someone who will beat you black and blue just because he thinks his meal is not cooked exactly right.

Inter-generational sex is another factor spreading the epidemic in many parts of the world and is often also driven by poverty. Young women see older men (it's usually that way round) as a ticket to a better life and with few other income-generating prospects available, engage in relationships with 'sugar daddies' who pay their school fees and keep them and their families fed and clothed. Many young women get involved in casual sex for the same reason. While girls in other parts of the world worry about their school reports and fall in love with images of pop stars, an 11-year-old South African girl describes life with a poignant adult worldliness: 'Sometimes girls go to *shebeens* [bars], look for people that they think have got money and go away with them. No one talks to the girl; the mother does not stop her. As long as the girl brings shopping bags along when she comes back, that becomes the end of the story.'

Sex-trafficking, migrancy and unemployment

AIDS has added a new dimension to sex work as many clients seek younger women thinking they will avoid

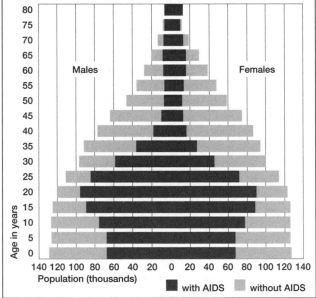

Dying in the prime of life

Before AIDS, most deaths clustered around early childhood and late adulthood. Now the epidemic is cutting a swathe through the most economically productive age groups. The impact will be felt deeply on the economy as well as on future generations, with many children raised without one or both parents.

Projected population structure with and without AIDS epidemic, Botswana, 2020

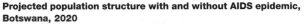

UNAIDS 2000. www.unaids.org

infection. There is speculation that the myth that sex with a virgin will cure AIDS is responsible for this. It is a myth that has surfaced in parts of Africa as well as Asia. However, there is no real evidence yet that this is encouraging sex with younger women. There is a growing concern that raising awareness of the myth is inadvertently promoting it, as well as further stigmatizing PWAs as willfully infecting others. More research clearly needs to be done in this area. However, it is a reality that younger girl children are being forced into sex and sex work. In many parts of Asia, trafficking of children and women is on the increase and is related to poverty and the expansion of tourism.

Poverty and unemployment – on the rise as a result of globalization and structural adjustment programs – compel many people to take work wherever they can find it, often long distances from home.

In Latin America, highly concentrated land ownership also forces large numbers of people, mostly men, to migrate in search of work. And HIV/AIDS spreads rapidly in the context of migrant labor. Far from home and loved ones for long periods, often in single-sex hostels with little access to recreational facilities, many such laborers seek comfort in casual sex with sex-workers or multiple partners. Poor access to information on HIV/AIDS and protection put both the men and the women at risk of contracting HIV. Come the end of the year, when it is time to take annual leave, the workers return to their wives, often carrying the lethal virus. Their wives, themselves vulnerable through lack of information and their status as women, are either unaware of the danger about to befall them, or if informed, may not have the power within the relationship to insist on condom use or other forms of safer sex. Recent research also suggests that in some instances, it is the wives who have become infected through their own sexual encounters during the husbands' long absences.

These factors are central in powering the epidemic in southern Africa and other regions as well as Latin America where one in every six families is unable to meet their basic needs.[5] Millions of children in that region live on the street often selling sex to survive. Not surprisingly, the epidemic is concentrated in these communities.

Countries in conflict and transition

War and persecution also play a part in the spread of HIV, contributing to high mobility with more than 100 million people moving between countries annually. Such great movement of people makes it difficult to contain the virus.

In countries that have recently experienced conflict or transition, a range of additional forces emerges. In Russia for example the mix of poverty, rising unem-ployment and subsequent despondency is feeding a heroin habit that is placing the country on the brink of an AIDS epidemic as virus transmission begins to travel into the general population. Drug-trafficking is on the increase in many Eastern European countries whose borders have been opened in recent years, post-conflict.

Africa, however, is living with the legacy of the slave trade and the subsequent scramble for Africa which created artificial borders and pitted societies against each other in the 'divide and rule' politics of colo-nization. Impoverishment of local populations to enrich the imperial powers and the placing of puppet dictators during the Cold War era to protect the West's interests have resulted in many dysfunctional states and widespread poverty. As a direct result too, the last 50 years have seen half of sub-Saharan Africa involved in wars and conflicts which uprooted millions of peo-ple. Armed conflict increases vulnerability to AIDS also because of sexual violence, often used as a weapon of war. This was most recently documented in Bosnia and Rwanda.

In Africa south of the Sahara, the presence of a more virulent strain of the virus (subclade HIV-1) has combined with these factors to make ripe conditions for the epidemic's spread.

The destruction of social structures and cultural systems in Africa and other parts of the world, through wars, social dislocation, migration and urbanization has also resulted in a breakdown of mores regulating sexual practice. Rites of passage into adulthood provided opportunities to educate the youth around matters of sexuality.

Understandably also, the insecurity provoked by war supersedes fears of a relatively distant death from a viral infection.

Deep in debt

Poverty and ill health have been entrenched through the debt trap. In many instances, poor countries pay more servicing their debt than they do on social services; most African governments spend up to three times more on debt repayments than on health care.[6] At the end of 1998, annual debt service payments from sub-Saharan Africa, the world's poorest region, to the richest countries amounted to $15.2 billion or 15 per cent of exports. The total debt currently stands at $231 billion.[7] In order to repay this, governments have been forced to borrow more from the International Monetary Fund (IMF), accepting punitive IMF and World Bank conditions for the rescheduling of payments. These conditions include structural adjustment policies (SAPs) – now renamed 'Poverty Reduction Strategies' – and currency devaluations that have led to deeper debt. The burden of repayment has been placed on poor people who are forced to pay for basic services that under international law are the right of everyone. Far from resuscitating economies, these programs have deepened poverty through the privatization of state enterprises with the concomitant shedding of jobs, and trade liberalization with declining tariffs and opening economies to foreign competition. They also invariably result in social spending cuts for health, welfare and education, increasing illiteracy and limiting access to information, and in this way contribute to spreading the virus (see also chapter 5).

User fees for basic health services (part of the SAPs package) have resulted in a dramatic decline in clinic attendance, exacerbating already high levels of morbidity and mortality and creating a time bomb in the context of this epidemic. In Kenya, for example, the World Bank insisted that clinics should charge a user fee of $2.15 for a basic examination to detect sexually transmitted infections (STIs). The presence of STIs has been shown to increase the risk of HIV transmission and the treatment of these infections remains one of the cornerstones of best practice approaches to HIV prevention. Clinic attendance in Kenya fell in some cases by as much as 60 per cent.[8]

Why poverty makes it worse

Conditions of poverty lead to poor nutrition and exposure to other illnesses, which often become chronic. This compromises the immune system and reduces the body's ability to fight off the HIV virus. Limited access to health services compounds this problem.

As well as increasing vulnerability to HIV infection, poverty also impacts on the course of the disease in HIV-positive people. Lack of food makes them weak and contributes to the rapid erosion of the immune system and hence earlier onset of AIDS. Without access to adequate health care, people who are HIV-positive are less likely to get treated promptly (if at all) for opportunistic infections and are more likely to succumb to them.

Being poor also limits people's access to treatment. In many countries, the cost of providing overpriced antiretroviral treatment would exceed the entire national health budget. In Northern countries, the use of drug therapy and breastmilk substitutes has virtually eliminated the pediatric AIDS epidemic. In many Southern countries by contrast, HIV-positive mothers are advised to continue breastfeeding since the lack of access to clean water (to wash bottles and mix powdered milk with) means the risk of their children dying from diarrhea and dehydration through bottle-feeding is still higher than the risk of transmission of HIV through breastmilk. The cost of formula milk and the drugs are also obstacles in poor countries.

Where countries or projects have been able to bring treatment to poor people, poverty can affect the efficacy of such treatment. Many of the drugs used to combat AIDS and opportunistic infections need to be taken with food to be effective – impossible in many parts of food-scarce or famine-stricken Africa.

AIDS exacerbates poverty

In turn, AIDS makes poverty worse. The epidemic hits the economically active strata of societies (see graphic **Bad for business**). The average life expectancy in sub-Saharan Africa for example has dropped from 62 years to around 47 years, according to UNAIDS. Households experience further poverty or destitution through loss of income as breadwinners become sick or die of AIDS. A UN Food and Agriculture

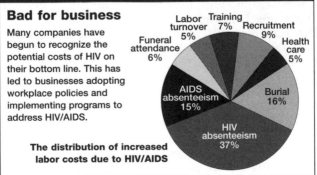

Bad for business

Many companies have begun to recognize the potential costs of HIV on their bottom line. This has led to businesses adopting workplace policies and implementing programs to address HIV/AIDS.

The distribution of increased labor costs due to HIV/AIDS

Labor turnover 5%
Training 7%
Recruitment 9%
Health care 5%
Funeral attendance 6%
AIDS absenteeism 15%
Burial 16%
HIV absenteeism 37%

M Roberts, B Rau, A Emery, 'Private Sector AIDS Policy: Businesses Managing AIDS. A Guide for Managers' (Arlington, VA: Family Health International AIDSCAP 1996) www.fhi.org/en/aids/aidscap/aidspub/policy/psapp. Cited in: T Barnett, A Whiteside, AIDS in the Twenty-First Century: Disease and Globalization (Palgrave Macmillan 2002).

Organization (FAO) study shows that the cost of caring for a family member with HIV/AIDS and paying for the funeral expenses when that person dies exceeds the average annual farm income. To make ends meet, rural households, already desperately poor, sell their productive assets such as livestock and land.

By 1999 over 13 million children had lost their parents to AIDS. As with so many other statistics, the majority of these – 95 per cent – were in sub-Saharan Africa. Many children from rural households, whose livelihoods are dependent on agriculture, are losing their parents before learning how to farm or take care of themselves. A study conducted by FAO in Namibia showed that half of the informants had left their land fallow due to labor shortages resulting from HIV/AIDS.[9]

In this way AIDS is contributing to an existing crisis of food shortage and famine in Africa, particularly – again – south of the Sahara.

According to the UNAIDS 2002 AIDS Report, by 2010, per capita GDP in some countries may drop by 8 per cent with heavily affected countries losing more than 20 per cent by 2020. Already, this region is said to have experienced a 2-4 per cent decrease in economic growth because of AIDS. This scenario is increasing the risk profile for investment.

As noted, poverty and AIDS are mutually reinforcing. AIDS specialists Tony Barnett and Alan Whiteside sum it up: 'The origins and the impact of a disease epidemic such as HIV/AIDS are linked at the root – they only appear to be different plants. The conditions that facilitate rapid spread of an infectious disease are also by and large those that make it hard for societies to respond, and ensure that its impact will be severe.'[10]

(ii) Women's new triple oppression

This next section explores the way women's vulnerability in society makes them vulnerable to the disease. 'I think this [AIDS] is the punishment we [as women] have been given because of our mother Eve, because she is the first lady who has made a mistake in the world and God has said to us we will suffer for that until we die. If she wasn't having that apple, in that garden, maybe we'd be having a good life.'[11]

While not everyone will agree with this young woman's explanation, there can be no doubt that women are bearing the brunt of the AIDS epidemic. It used to be said that black, poor, women faced a triple oppression (of race, class and gender). Now, AIDS makes their load even heavier. Firstly, they are biologically more vulnerable to infection. Secondly, their unequal standing in relation to men makes them less able to protect themselves against the disease. Thirdly, as the epidemic takes root and more people are in need of care, women nurse sick relatives, children and members of their community. Many girls are forced to drop out of school to look after the household, their siblings and ill parents. When the parents die, it is the girls who usually take over. In many countries this is affecting the lives of a substantial number of young women. In Swaziland for example, UNAIDS notes that school enrolment has fallen by 36 per cent – mostly of girls – as a result of the epidemic.

Biological vulnerability

A woman's body structure makes her at least twice as likely to contract HIV from an infected man. This is because she is the receptive sex partner and infected semen stays in the vagina for a considerable time after sex, giving the virus more opportunity to enter the bloodstream. Any cuts or sores in the vaginal wall greatly increase the risk as the HIV then has direct access to her blood. These sores can result from

In sub-Saharan Africa alone, an estimated 12.2 million women carry the virus compared with 10.1 million men. In some countries, girls are 5-6 times more likely to be infected than teenage boys. ∎

Sexual coercion

Almost a third of young women aged 15-19 in KwaZulu Natal, South Africa, associate their first sexual encounter with some form of coercion. Their ability to negotiate safer sex in this context is obviously severely compromised.

Reported experiences of first sexual experiences

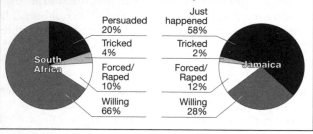

South Africa		Jamaica	
Persuaded	20%	Just happened	58%
Tricked	4%	Tricked	2%
Forced/Raped	10%	Forced/Raped	12%
Willing	66%	Willing	28%

sexually transmitted infections to cancer of the cervix or from 'rough' or violent sex. Poor lubrication due to age, biology or lack of adequate foreplay can also make them more susceptible to tears in the vaginal wall during sex, increasing the chance of infection.

Gender inequality

Gender is a society's way of defining the roles and responsibilities of men and women. It is a societal construct that has never been great for women and, in the context of AIDS, is also proving detrimental to men. Almost without exception, societies and cultures across the world groom men into a masculinity that celebrates multiple sexual partners and heterosexuality. This puts young boys and men under pressure to have sex and lots of it, placing them at risk of sexually transmitted infections including HIV/AIDS. It also means that men having sex with men (MSM) are less likely to reveal their homosexual orientation, making access to life-protecting information and services difficult. Part of the masculine identity encourages risk-taking which often leads to substance abuse, including alcohol and drugs (of course women do these too). This can result in impaired judgment in the heat of the moment, when hard choices need to be made – for example deciding not to use a condom or having sex even if a condom is not available.

According to health economist Lesley Doyal, 'growing up male' involves the need to be seen as 'hard' which can lead to an unwillingness to admit vulnerability. This may prevent many men from taking health promotion messages seriously and from consulting a doctor when problems arise.[12]

As seen earlier, societal notions of masculinity also preclude and therefore stigmatize men who have sex with men and many remain 'in the closet', leading external lives of 'heterosexuality'. This stops them from seeking help and has resulted in 'hidden' epidemics throughout the world. As many such men may also be having sex with women, the epidemic proliferates. Many people, totally unbiased by fact, believe that homosexuality does not exist in certain cultures and in numerous countries it has been criminalized. In these and other places where heterosexual transmission is the dominant means of spread, prevention programs targeting men who have sex with men are often, unfortunately, absent.

Despite the increased male vulnerability as a result of gender constructs, according to the June 2001 UN Special Session on HIV/AIDS in most societies girls and women face higher risks of HIV infection than men because their diminished economic and social status compromises their ability to choose safer and healthier life strategies. Geeta Rao Gupta of the International Center for Research on Women (ICRW), a nonprofit institute in Washington DC, points out that 'in most societies women are perceived as being responsible for reproductive and productive tasks within the home and men are seen as being responsible primarily for the productive tasks outside the home. Because of that stereotyping, women have less access to resources outside the home – education, employment, land, income, credit, mobility – that in most societies give individuals power. That imbalance of power in the social and economic spheres of life translates into a power imbalance in heterosexual relationships. As a result, men, more often than women, are able to control where, when and how sex takes place.'[13]

For women the combination of patriarchy and gender inequality (and consequent gender violence), poverty, and female biological vulnerability is lethal. In sub-Saharan Africa alone, an estimated 12.2 million women carry the virus compared with 10.1 million men. In some countries, girls are 5-6 times more likely to be infected than teenage boys.[14] According to a recent UN Development Program report: 'The sex ratios of men and women living with HIV/AIDS is not just a game of numbers. It is essentially an issue of gender-power relations. There is now a fast-growing understanding that gender inequality heightens women's vulnerability to the epidemic and leaves them with untenable burdens when HIV/AIDS enters households and communities.'

Around the world, inequality limits millions of women's access to basic health services and so to life-saving prevention information, treatment for sexually transmitted infections or opportunistic infections related to AIDS. When family resources are low, men are also more likely than women to be sent for or admitted to healthcare when they are sick. Although in the UK the National Health Service removed financial obstacles to healthcare access, according to British health economist Lesley Doyal there is still evidence that women are treated by some doctors as less valuable than men. Doyal maintains that the impact of this discrimination reaches beyond demeaning attitudes to include the unequal allocation of clinical resources.[15]

'You're too young'

Young women – the very group in which the epidemic is spreading most rapidly – are particularly affected by health professionals' attitudes that are in turn influenced by gender socialization. Young women often find it difficult to use reproductive health services for fear of censure. Stories abound of them being turned away, told they are too young to be thinking of sex or are blamed and made to feel 'dirty' or 'sinful' for having a sexually transmitted infection. Especially in smaller communities, confidentiality becomes an issue, as the health worker may well know the girl's family.

One of the major ways in which gender inequality places women at risk is by preventing them from having a say in the terms and circumstances of sex. In this context, the 'ABC' (Abstain, Be faithful, wear a Condom) approach to AIDS prevention – the mainstay of most prevention programs – has proven over-simplistic. As we have seen, women are often in no position to bargain with men. Many are not at liberty to insist on fidelity from their partner and it is almost impossible to negotiate any form of protection with a man who believes that it is his right to expect his lover's unquestioning obedience. This obedience is

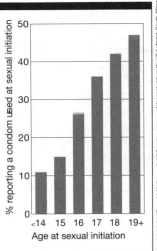

Young at heart, high at risk

Many young people throughout the world are having sex at an age where they do not have the knowledge, skills or power to negotiate safer sex. The chances of condoms being used increases with age. Delaying the age of sexual onset therefore, is an important strategy to protect youth.

Percentage of adolescent girls in KwaZulu Natal, South Africa who report a condom being used at first sexual intercourse, by age at sexual initiation, 1999

Manzini, Ntaki, 'Sexual initiation and childbearing among adolescent girls in KwaZulu Natal, South Africa', Reproductive Health Matters, 9 (17): May 2001. Cited in: 'Young People and HIV/AIDS "Opportunity in Crisis', UNICEF, UNAIDS, WHO, 2002. www.unaids.org

South Africa has the dubious honor of being the rape capital of the world. It is reckoned that a woman is raped every 17 seconds. When this is linked with the fact that 1 in every 9 South Africans is HIV-positive, the consequences are catastrophic. ∎

often enforced through physical violence or the fear of it. Abstinence is difficult to uphold as a lifestyle choice in the context of rape and the widespread belief that coerced sex by boyfriends or husbands does not constitute rape.

The UN session on HIV/AIDS pointed to the growing evidence that a large share of new cases of HIV infection is due to gender-based violence in homes, schools, the workplace and other social spheres. In addition, in settings of civil disorder and war, women and girls are often systematically targeted for abuse (including sexual abuse). As a Ugandan woman lamented: 'During times of war, soldiers took money and sometimes killed men, but always they took money and sex from women.'[16]

Internationally, gender-based violence is increasingly recognized as a public health priority. A recent study has estimated that 19 per cent of the total disease burden carried by women aged 15-44 in developed countries is the result of domestic violence and rape.[17] Perhaps most deadly is the convergence of the high incidence of rape in countries with soaring rates of HIV infection. South Africa, for example, has the dubious honor of being the rape capital of the world. While people squabble about the figures, at the last count a woman is raped every 17 seconds. Couple this with the fact that 1 in every 9 South Africans is HIV-positive and you have a recipe for disaster. The story of 30-year-old Joyce Malope, a Johannesburg AIDS activist, infected with the virus after a brutal encounter, is not uncommon (see box).

While rape by strangers is commonplace, more women are infected by their partners under circumstances where violence or fear of it determines how and when sex occurs. According to the UN, up to 80 per cent of cases where women in long-term relationships are HIV-positive, they acquired the virus from their partners. This takes place in a context where the male prerogative to multiple sexual partners is often the 'accepted' norm. Frighteningly, marriage is one of the greatest risk factors for women today.

Patriarchy and female subordination

In many countries the problem is rooted in a patriarchal society that subordinates women. According to Karen Dzumbira of Women in Law and Development in Africa (WiLDAF), cultural systems are all too often used to legitimize men's rights over women. Violence is often condoned or tolerated as a way of maintaining control. In the HIV/AIDS pandemic, cultural practices can be a double-edged sword. Some aspects, such as male circumcision, have been shown to be protective, and positive practices have been successfully used to promote prevention (see chapter 5). However,

Joyce Malope's story

I was walking home from work when he drove up to me. He was dressed as a priest, soft spoken and sweet. There was even a bible on the seat of his car. I said, 'Father, how can I help you?' He asked directions to a church he was visiting. It was close to my place. I thought to myself, why shouldn't I help this priest, only to find later, he was going to be my rapist...

En route, another guy jumped inside. He pulled out a gun and said 'If you scream I'm going to kill you.' They put a plastic bag over my head. All I could see was lights. He raped me the whole night. He put the gun into my mouth. At the time, I didn't think of HIV, I just thought, 'as long as you don't kill me.'

After they were finished, they dropped me on the pavement near my place. I kept on passing out. No one stopped to help. I heard people say 'maybe she was beaten up by her husband. Probably he found her sleeping with someone else'. Like that justified anything. Finally a man stopped and took me to hospital. My first HIV test was negative. I was told to come back after the window period [the period during which one is infected but the virus is not yet detectable through antibodies in the blood]. It was then that I found out I was positive. ∎

other cultural aspects in both the North and South place women at great risk. These range from female genital circumcision or cutting, wife inheritance (where a woman must marry her late husband's brother), to bride price. 'The *lobola* system (bride price in South Africa) reinforces the idea that a woman is a man's property and he can do with her what he wishes,' says Karen Dzumbira. Some argue that *lobola* is intended as a positive way of cementing a relationship between two families but according to Joyce Malope the reality for many men is: 'I've paid money for you... If I say jump – you jump.'

Female genital circumcision is another form of violence against women that is contributing to the spread of AIDS. In an attempt to take into account the feelings of women who choose to undergo the practice it is often referred to as female genital 'cutting'. Others, arguing to 'call a spade a spade' prefer the term 'female genital mutilation'. Whatever the name, it makes women more vulnerable to AIDS. The practice is widespread in countries such as Egypt (97 per cent of women), Mali (94 per cent) and Sudan (89 per cent)[18] and many more. The process means women's external genitalia are surgically altered – sometimes with a knife which if not sterilized properly can play a role in transmitting HIV or other infections. The degree of cutting varies from removal of the *labia majora* to infibulation. This involves removing the entire vulval tissue including the clitoris and the *labia majora* and *minora*. The wound is closed leaving a tiny opening the size of a matchstick – enough to allow the escape of urine and menstrual blood but obviously not enough to allow penetration. The intention is to keep the woman 'chaste' for her future husband. He has to forcibly enter her, inevitably leading to tears (both kinds) and often major bleeding. You don't need to be a rocket scientist to see the risk of HIV transmission under these circumstances.

Women are also vulnerable because many cultures

place such a high premium on fertility as a reflection of wealth. As a result, millions of women are placed in an impossible situation where, under tremendous pressure to have children, they are reluctant or unable to insist on condom use.

The trap of abuse

Societal constructs of what constitutes a 'good girl' also intimidate women from self-protection. Joyce Malope explains that 'men take you as "sluts" if you ask them to wear a condom. They'll ask you why you are acting like a prostitute. They accuse you of sleeping around or they say, "You don't trust me". Some will just beat you up. When it comes to using a condom, men complain they won't "eat a sweet with its wrapper on".'

A further injustice is the belief that vaginal lubrication signifies infidelity. To avoid the real threat of violent punishment or to please men who favor a 'tighter' vagina, many women insert herbs and other substances inside their vaginas to 'dry up'. Dry sex makes vaginal abrasion more likely and increases the risk of HIV transmission if their partner carries the virus.

Dependent on men for financial support, many women are trapped in abusive relationships that expose them to HIV infection. The way Joyce describes it, 'If he is supporting you, you have to listen to him – your choice is to stay and get beaten or he leaves. [To cover up] women will say they were beaten by thugs – to survive, you end up protecting the very person who is killing you.' The relationship is perpetuated through generations. 'Boys see our fathers doing it, so they take it as normal. Even our mums will say, "If he beats you, try to change your attitude". Our mums want us to do the same as they did, whereas now it's the new millennium.'

South African Catholic Bishop Kevin Dowling was so moved by the plight of women with regard to AIDS that he tried (unsuccessfully) to overturn the Church's ban on condom use there. 'What prompted me to take a different position has come out of anguished reflection of several years… of years of walking with people experiencing death in appalling situations of poverty, particularly experiencing the reality on the ground for so many women who are disadvantaged socially, economically and culturally – women who have very little say over their lives; women who are in abusive relationships; women who through desperate poverty are forced into liaisons in search of simply how to survive until tomorrow morning.' The official response was unsympathetic. One priest replied: 'If you are going save a life by using an immoral means, I don't think you are actually saving a life.'[19]

Circle of violence

Just as violence against women is a contributory factor in the spread of HIV, so the epidemic increases levels of violence against women. Ironically, because many women learn of their HIV status only when pregnant, they are the ones accused of 'bringing AIDS home'. With violence or rejection a common consequence, most women will not reveal that they are HIV-positive to their partners. In a recent study of women attending a health clinic in Dar es Salaam, Tanzania, fear of violence and abandonment was cited as the main reason for not saying they were infected. Nearly 39 per cent said that they had been physically abused by a partner and about 17 per cent had been sexually abused. In Kenya, more than half of a group of HIV-positive women hid the news from their partners for similar reasons.[20]

For Sowetan-born Thembane the consequences of disclosure were bleak: 'When I told my husband he said, "You are lying". He beat me in my face, because of the HIV thing. He didn't want me to say anything to him or anyone else. I continued to speak about it though, because it worries me and I think about my life and my child and family.' Thembane's husband refused to go for a test and eventually left her.

The AIDS epidemic is shrouded in stigma and fear (see next section). Revealing that one is HIV-positive is often perceived as 'bringing shame' on families and communities. So many women remain silent and don't seek the help they need to stay healthy. Fear of beatings or rape and being labeled a 'bad girl' prevents women from going for voluntary testing and seeking counseling or treatment. According to female African delegates at an international AIDS conference, women have to run a gauntlet of taboo, male opposition and financial worry to get access to HIV tests and drugs. These hurdles are also making it difficult for pregnant women to take steps to prevent transmission to their children. While some seek treatment 'under cover', they then later have to explain to the fathers why they are not breastfeeding (see next chapter on the transmission of HIV through breastmilk).

Centuries of gender socialization are obviously not easy to reverse but historically, societies have changed when the need is stark. The ICRW's Gupta sums this up: 'I don't believe that culture is immutable. We have seen the norms of male and female roles change over our own lifetime. In the West, during and after the Second World War, women's roles changed because society needed women – like Rosie the Riveter – to step up and play a different role, at least for a short period of time. That experience planted the seeds of change.'[21]

It is clear that until gender inequality is removed, AIDS will proliferate.

(iii) Stigma – when being positive can be negative

This third section examines the problem of stigmatizing people with AIDS. Dominic D'Souza, one of the first people openly living with HIV in India, was employed by the Goa branch of the World Wide Fund for Nature (WWF). A regular blood donor, when his HIV-positive status was discovered D'Souza was held at a TB sanatorium under armed guard. No-one touched him and food was left at the door of the cell. After 64 days he was released but only as a result of demonstrations and protest marches organized by his family and friends. Adding insult to injury, he was subsequently fired from WWF. Dominic became an outspoken activist protesting stigma until his death in May 1992.[22]

Spin the globe and select any country in the world and you will find similar stories of discrimination based on a person's HIV status. In Swaziland prominent politicians proposed that people with HIV/AIDS (PWAs) should be forced to wear identification badges and be herded into special segregated areas where they would not be able to contaminate 'normal people'.[23]

In the Californian elections of November 1986, the draconian Proposition 64 was voted upon and thankfully defeated by a two-thirds majority. However, one third of the voters actually supported this legislation that would prevent HIV-positive people from being employed as teachers, employees or students in public or private schools, or as commercial food handlers. In

Gugu Dlamini's story

Across the road from the vast International Convention Center in Durban, South Africa – host to the 13th International Conference on AIDS – is a little park dedicated to the memory of Gugu Dlamini. Sitting on the benches amidst the green grass and flowers, it is hard to imagine the terrible act of cruelty that led to Gugu's murder on 12 December 1998. An AIDS activist in the sprawling Durban township of KwaMashu, Gugu took a brave decision when she stepped up onto a public platform to tell people that she was HIV-positive. Her motivation was pure and simple – to create more openness about the disease, to break the silence and the stigma that envelops it. By making a simple statement – that she, Gugu Dlamini, a person like you and me – could become HIV-positive, Gugu's hope was that other ordinary people would wake up and start to see themselves as also at risk; that AIDS is not something that happens to 'other' people. How ironic therefore that shortly after returning home from the meeting, Gugu was attacked by her neighbors, accusing her of bringing shame on their community. She was beaten to death. ■

1998, an 8-year-old girl was refused admission to a Girl Scout troop in the New York area on the grounds that she was HIV-positive.

New York ACT UP activist Eric Sawyer describes how he and his emaciated partner, who had noticeable Kaposi's Sarcoma on his face, were confronted by a hostile, homophobic public in restaurants with comments like: 'You diseased faggots, why don't you go somewhere else and die.'[24] People have been – and continue to be – thrown out of their homes by their families, fired from their work and shunned by their communities. In 1986, a spokesperson for the Belgian Ministry of Health announced its intent to implement compulsory HIV testing for African students with the following statement: 'The Belgian Government wants to warn these countries that it has no need to invest money and to invest time in these students who are ill, sick and after some years, dead.'[25] Ironically, while the West blamed Africa for AIDS, China blames the West for 'bringing homosexuality and injecting drug use to Asia' and AIDS or 'aizibing' is referred to by some as 'loving capitalism disease'.[26]

Shame and stigma reinforce the silence around HIV/AIDS and present one of the major obstacles to global efforts to defeat the epidemic. Silence perpetuates myths that reinforce the stigma and lead to more silence. Stigma manifests in the reluctance of people to test for the virus and receive early treatment and care. It pushes the epidemic underground, preventing people from telling those close to them and in so doing, denying themselves the support they need to remain healthy. It stops pregnant women taking medication that could prevent transmission to their children and it makes people shun preventive information that could save lives. Sadly, stigma results in many families refusing to take care of the children whose parents have died of AIDS, leading to a great increase in the number of young children heading households.

In the US, the Ray family with three HIV-positive sons with hemophilia moved from Florida to Alabama after the children were refused entry to school. The move brought no respite to the discrimination. The children were again refused school entry and the family home was torched by an arsonist. ■

Stigma, discrimination and human rights

HIV-related discrimination has been described by UNAIDS as 'action that results from stigma. It occurs when a distinction is made against a person that results in their being treated unfairly and unjustly on the basis of their actual or presumed HIV status or their belonging, or being perceived to belong to a particular group. It results in rejection, denial and discrediting, and consequently leads to discrimination, which inevitably leads to the violation of human rights'.[28] AIDS stigma is expressed around the world in different ways including ostracism, discrimination, rejection and avoidance of people living with HIV/AIDS, compulsory HIV testing without prior consent or protection of confidentiality, violence against people who are perceived to have AIDS or to be HIV-positive and quarantine of persons with HIV.[29]

Around the world AIDS has brought out the best and the worst of us: from the murder of Gugu Dlamini (see box) to the bravery of Dominic D'Souza and the parents who have overcome their own homophobia to become loving and supportive caregivers of their gay children living with HIV/AIDS.

Myths of HIV transmission

But what is it about HIV/AIDS that has brought out our darkest side? First off, it is the fact that the disease is incurable and before the advent of antiretrovirals (ARVs), led inevitably to a premature death. For most of the world, where ARVs are beyond the price range of the average person or national health budget, this remains largely the case. Throughout the ages humanity has responded to incurable diseases with fear and discrimination. Lepers in the Dark Ages of Europe were compelled – on pain of death – to warn everyone of their illness by ringing a bell and shouting out 'unclean' whenever they appeared in public. During the great plague that swept Europe in the 1660s, people looked for scapegoats. Jews were accused of bribing lepers to poison the city wells and the roots of later atrocities committed against the Jews can be traced back, in part, to this period. While civilization may have advanced, we have not necessarily elevated ourselves. Our response to HIV/AIDS is proof enough.

Fear and discrimination are the offspring of stigma and have their base in ignorance and lack of information. Much of the hysteria around AIDS for example, stems from the erroneous belief that the virus can be transmitted through casual contact such as from sneezes, touching or sharing cutlery with an infected person. Even the Mass has been tainted with some people refraining from drinking from a common chalice. It is this fear that has led to incidents in America and Australia and other parts of the world, such as banning HIV-positive children from school.

A US study found that in 1999, 30 per cent of people polled would feel uncomfortable having their children attend school with another child who is HIV-positive and over one-fifth would feel uncomfortable around an office co-worker with HIV. While the proportion of those who felt afraid of people with HIV declined from 35 per cent in 1991, the numbers were still frighteningly high at one in five. The study found that mistaken beliefs about the mechanisms of HIV transmission were widespread and that these beliefs were highest among those people most likely to discriminate against PWAs. Almost 20 years into the epidemic, 41 per cent still believed they could get AIDS from using public toilets and half those interviews believed they could get AIDS from being coughed on by an infected person. About half of those surveyed believed they could get

AIDS by sharing a drinking glass. Almost 30 per cent of respondents said they would avoid shopping at a neighborhood grocery store if they knew the owner was HIV-positive.[30] This misinformation was found to have increased since 1991. The study also found that growing numbers of Americans now blame PWAs themselves for their own illness.

Pointing the finger

Much of this blame has to do with the fact that HIV/AIDS is associated with sex and was first profiled in already marginalized and stigmatized communities such as gay men, sex-workers, injecting drug users and people having sex with multiple partners. It also may have something to do with the global focus of preventive programs on personal responsibility. While this is an understandable tack – we all need to take responsibility for our actions – it belies the fact that for millions of people this degree of personal control over one's life and environment is not easy. Take for example the countless people who become HIV-positive after being raped or the women who have no power to negotiate safer sex within their relationships. Even this argument however, lends itself dangerously toward the division of the world into those who are 'innocent', and those who are 'guilty' and so by implication 'deserve' to get HIV/AIDS. Children are often referred to as the epidemic's 'innocent victims' implying that their mothers who transmitted the virus to them are somehow guilty. Infected sex-workers and gays are described as 'getting their just desserts'. The epidemic has been described as 'part of God's plan to rid the world of sinners'. In such a world, the 'innocents' need to be protected from the 'guilty'.

'I'm not ashamed. I have the virus and I want to stop as many people as I can from sharing my fate. Ignoring the problem will only make it worse.' ■

Sergei, former intravenous drug user, Russia.

The fact that HIV/AIDS first gained prominence amongst homosexual men in North America has meant that much of the world's venom has been directed at the gay community. Ironically, at a UN session on human rights and AIDS in June 2001, a group of religious participants blackballed the participation of Karyn Kaplan of the International Gay and Lesbian Human Rights Commission. A resolution was introduced at the General Assembly to allow Kaplan to participate. Alarmingly, almost a third of the UN member nations were willing to boycott the vote and derail the entire session.[31]

The media has fed the frenzy of discrimination against minorities and groups perceived somehow to be 'deviant'. Take these headlines in a 1989 edition of the London *News of the World*: 'The House That Died of Shame'. The article reports: 'The specter of AIDS-ravaged film star Rock Hudson is finally being exorcised from the mansion he once used as a gay pleasure palace.'[32] The association of 'gayness' with 'decadence and promiscuity' that led to Hudson's AIDS status is but one example of how the media has continuously characterized it as a gay disease linked to a gay lifestyle that is synonymous with 'deviance'.

The media also uses language and photographs that incite public fear and paranoia. Words such as 'plague' (usually 'gay plague') and images of authorities burning the automobile of an accident victim infected with HIV or police wearing yellow rubber gloves while arresting gay protestors only serve to endorse public fear and misunderstanding.[33] Note how Hudson's spirit is referred to as having been 'exorcised' from his house. Being gay and having AIDS are equated seamlessly with sin. Like the devil, Hudson's spirit had to be driven out as something evil.

Religion

Religion is often ambivalent in its views of PWAs. While many religious mores promote protection, care and support, religions have also sadly fanned the flames of discrimination. The association of HIV/AIDS with behaviors that may be forbidden by religious or traditional teachings such as pre-and extra-marital sex, sex work, or men having sex with men has provided fuel for priests delivering fire and brimstone sermons across the globe, making HIV/AIDS synonymous with sin and 'divine punishment' in the minds of many.

While the science of transmission may be well understood (see next chapter), people still seek reasons to explain why, in the lottery where only some get infected, it happened to them. Spiritual interpretations provide much sought-after explanations for their misfortunes.

Perpetuating inequalities

As noted, the linking of an incurable disease with sex – already a taboo subject in many parts of the world – adds to the silence around HIV/AIDS, reinforcing the myths that perpetuate the stigma. It's a vicious circle that drives the epidemic out of sight, stopping people from disclosing and seeking help for fear of being labeled as someone 'bad' or 'sinful'. As we have seen, the sitgma associated with HIV/AIDS feeds inequalities of gender, sexuality, class and race.

HIV/AIDS divides humanity into 'them and us' and this is one of the most dangerous repercussions of stigma. Ironically, despite the fact that the epidemic is largely spread through heterosexual sex in most parts of the world, characterizations of HIV/AIDS as a 'gay' disease persist. Many white people see it as a 'black disease'; many black people see it as a disease of 'white gay men'. The irony is that the 'us' who discriminate may well be 'them' but don't know it yet, because they have not been tested. The tragedy is that the stigma associated with HIV/AIDS will prevent many people from having a test. This 'othering' results in a low perception of personal risk. Lulled into a false sense of security, people engage in unsafe behavior. In a similar way, the association of HIV/AIDS with multiple sexual partners and the focussing of prevention campaigns on fidelity ironically has led many monogamous couples to perceive themselves as safe, without taking into account one's status before entering the current 'faithful' relationship.

A recent study in North America found that many people believe that there is a strong chance of contracting HIV during sex between two *uninfected* homosexual men and that HIV can be transmitted through injecting drugs per se, without actually sharing needles.[34] To lessen discrimination there has been a move away from categorizing groups as 'high risk' towards descriptions of 'high-risk behaviors'. Unprotected anal sex is a high-risk behavior. Being homosexual is not. Many heterosexual people have anal sex and if they do so unprotected they stand as much chance of contracting the virus from a partner with HIV as would a gay man.

Feeding into existing xenophobia, 'locals' blame 'foreigners' for 'bringing AIDS into their countries'. Some countries check travelers' HIV status and can refuse entry if they are HIV-positive. In 1986, the British House of Commons seriously debated the issue of whether there should be a ban on travel by Africans to the North or whether all Africans should submit blood tests for HIV at the point of immigration. Thankfully the motion was defeated.[35] Beyond the human rights violations involved in such restrictions, the idea of barricading any country against outside infection is patently ridiculous when almost every nation now has its own HIV/AIDS epidemic.

Voluntary testing and prevention

The world is increasingly recognizing that the stigma surrounding HIV/AIDS is retarding prevention, care and support efforts. Reluctance to go for voluntary testing is one of the many ways in which this manifests. Such testing is recognized as an important component of a country's response to the epidemic. Voluntary testing programs are coupled with pre- and post-test counseling which help prepare a person for either a positive or a negative result. The counseling provides an opportunity for education on how HIV is transmitted, helping protect those who are negative from future transmission. For those who are already positive, knowing this and how the virus is transmitted can help prevent the unwitting infection of others. Knowing one's status can also help one stay healthier longer through lifestyle modification and early treatment of opportunistic infections. Beyond the impact on the lives of the individuals concerned, early diagnosis and entry into the healthcare system have societal benefits too. These include reduced hospitalization costs and improved productivity. However, according to recent studies, two-thirds of gay and bisexual men in the US claimed that they had delayed testing because of the stigma surrounding the disease.[36] Many feared that their status would be revealed to others including employers, and that they would be ostracized or fired as a result.

Prejudice and homophobia continue to block education and outreach work. In 2001 four HIV/AIDS educators in Lucknow, India, working with men who have sex with men were arrested and allegedly tortured by police. They had been charged under Section 377 of the Indian Penal Code which outlaws 'carnal intercourse against the order of nature'. They were also charged for distributing HIV/AIDS education material under Section 292 which criminalizes the sale of 'obscene books'. Activist pressure helped secure their release after up to 45 days' imprisonment. Mr Bondyopadhyay, a lawyer working on the case said: 'The men were beaten, denied food, forced to drink sewer water, abused regularly and refused treatment when they got sick.'[37]

Ironically, health-workers – at the forefront of the epidemic – are also often at the forefront of discrimination. Stories abound of health-workers refusing to treat people with HIV and AIDS. A US survey found that health professionals preferred to care for patients who have acquired HIV through a blood transfusion rather than through any other route of transmission.[38]

Promoting human rights

Dealing with stigma has become a major focus of HIV/AIDS work. Strategies include encouraging both 'ordinary' and high-profile citizens to say when they are HIV-positive, as well as strengthening human rights mechanisms to combat discrimination. And as seen in chapter 1, in 1998 UNAIDS and the UN High Commissioner for Human Rights published their International Guidelines, a set of recommendations to member states on ways to prevent HIV/AIDS-related discrimination. The need to promote and protect human rights (see more on this in chapter 5) arose partially in response to the growing number of incidents of HIV/AIDS-related prejudice, including the rise of discriminatory legislation. It also arose in response to the fact that stigma reduces people's autonomy and ability to make protective choices, thereby increasing their personal risk as well as influencing the epidemiology of the epidemic.[39] Protecting the rights of people with HIV creates greater openness and more incentives to be tested, counseled and treated, safeguarding both themselves and others.

HIV/AIDS is different from diseases that are visible or highly infectious through casual contact (see chapter 3 on transmission), where protection of those who are uninfected may justify reasonable restrictions on those infected. Justice Michael Kirby, of the Australian Supreme Court, describes this as 'the AIDS paradox' whereby protecting the rights of people without HIV is best served through the protection of the rights of people who have HIV.

The epidemic impacts on the most fundamental aspects of human rights, including the rights of life and health as well as social and economic rights. These include the right to be protected from poverty and from gender-related discrimination.

HIV/AIDS has been described as the biggest ever human rights challenge for the international community. History has already judged the world harshly for its inadequate response to this crisis. While some progress is now being made, there is still a long way to go before that judgment will change.

1 P Farmer, *Infections and Inequalities: The Modern Plagues* (University of California Press 2001). **2** UNAIDS/WHO 2002, *AIDS epidemic update: December 2002*. **3** C Moller, 'House of Love', *Steps to the Future* television series, 2001. **4** UNAIDS/WHO 2002, *AIDS Epidemic Update: December 2002*. **5** 'Humanitarian Action: Latin American Regional Information', *Association François-Xavier Bagnoud* www.fxb.org/action/latinamer.html **6** Africa: Debt and AIDS, 06/02/02, http://www.sas.upenn.edu/African_Studies/Urgent_Action/apic-061402.html. **7** Jubilee 2000. http://www.jubilee2000uk.org/analysis/reports/needle.htm **8** W Ellwood, 'We all have AIDS', *New Internationalist*, No 346, June 2002. **9** Southern African Regional Poverty Network, *HSRC Poverty Briefing* No 2, September 2002. **10** T Barnett, and A Whiteside, *Aids in the Twenty-First Century: Disease and Globalization* (Palgrave Macmillan 2002). **11** Interview with South African women in M Emett, 'Body and Soul', *Steps to the Future* television series, 2001. **12** S Griffiths, 'Men's health: unhealthy lifestyles and unwillingness to seek medical help. *BMJ*, 312: 69-70, 1996. Cited in L Doyal, 'Sex, gender, and health: the need for a new approach', *BMJ*, 323: 1061-1063, November 2001. **13** A Kott, 'Gender and the epidemic', *Ford Foundation Report*, Summer 2002. **14** 'Fact sheet on Gender and HIV/AIDS', produced for the UNGASS Special Session on HIV/AIDS, June 2001, http://www.un.org/ga/aids/ungassfactsheets/html/fsgender_en.htm **15** L Doyal, *Women and health services* (Open University Press 1998). **16** T Barnett and A Whiteside, *Aids in the Twenty-First Century: Disease and Globalization* (Palgrave Macmillan 2002) p 136. **17** World Bank, *World Development Report 1993: investing in health*. (Oxford University Press, 1993). Cited in L Doyal, 'Sex, gender, and health: the need for a new approach', *BMJ*, 323: 1061-1063, November 2001. **18** National Demographic Health Surveys available from Macro International Inc. (http://www.measuredhs.int), Calverton, Maryland USA, cited on www.who.int/frh-whd/FGM/FGM%20prev%update.html **19** M Emmett, 'Body and Soul', *Steps for the Future* television series, 2001. **20** UNAIDS/WHO 2001, *AIDS Epidemic Update 2001*, cited in W Ellwood, 'We all have AIDS', *New Internationalist,* No 346, June 2002. **21** A Kott,

'Gender and the epidemic', *Ford Foundation Report*, Summer 2002. **22** A Row Kavi, D Godrej, 'Bigots take the temple', *New Internationalist*, No 250, December 1993. **23** L Masuku, 'Swaziland's AIDS Ambassador', *Africa Eye News Service*, August 2001, cited in W Ellwood, 'We all have AIDS', *New Internationalist* No 346, June 2002. **24** P Brooks, 'An Account of a Catastrophe Foretold', *Steps for the Future* television series, 2001. **25** P Brooks, op. cit. **26** *The Guardian*, 5 March 1990, p 10, cited on www.avert.org/his87-92.htm **27** 'So little time – a brief history of AIDS/HIV', www.aegis.com/topics/timeline/default.asp **28** Regional Consultation Meeting on Stigma and HIV/AIDS in Africa; 4-6 June 2001; Dar es Salaam, Tanzania. UNAIDS, Health & Development Networks and the Swedish International Development Agency (SIDA). www.unaids.org. **29** http://psychology. Ucdavis.edu/rainbow/html/aids.html accessed 04/09/2002 **30** GM Herek, JP Capitanio, KF Widaman, 'HIV-Related Stigma and Knowledge in the United States: Prevalence and trends, 1991-1999', *American Journal of Public Health*, 92 (3) 2002. **31** K Cogswell, 'Beating the Gay Stigma of AIDS', *The Gully*, www.thegully.com/essays/gaymundo/010628global_AIDS.html 04/09/2002 **32** *The Independent* (UK) 2 August 1989, cited in TW Netter, 'The Media and AIDS: A Global Perspective', chapter in 'Aids Prevention through Education: A World View'. Eds J Sepulveda, H Fineberg, J Mann (Oxford University Press 1992). **33** TW Netter, 'The Media and AIDS: A Global Perspective', chapter in J Sepulveda, H Fineberg, J Mann (Eds) *Aids Prevention through Education: A World View*, (Oxford University Press 1992). **34** *AIDS Action Policy Facts*, January 2001. www.aidsaction.com **35** 'Folk devils and moral panics: myths about AIDS', *New Internationalist*, No 169, March 1987. **36** *AIDS Action Policy Facts*, January 2001. www.aidsaction.com **37** www.iglhrc.org/news/press/pr_020408.html **38** *AIDS Action Policy Facts*, January 2001. www.aidsaction.com **39** M Heywood, 'HIV and AIDS: From the Perspective of Human Rights and Legal Protection', in 'One Step Further – Responses to HIV/AIDS', *Sida Studies* No 7, 2002.

3 Sex, drugs and rock'n'roll – the science of HIV

'I'm living a victorious life – I can't change the fact that I have AIDS, but I can change my attitude towards it. For me, contracting HIV hasn't been about dying, it's been about living. I appreciate every moment of my life. Having HIV has brought out the strong and dynamic woman in me.'[1]

Musa Njoko, South Africa.

If HIV was a person, it would be a nasty piece of work. Sneaky in many ways, it seems built for surviving today's mean streets. Although fragile and unable to live for long periods outside the human body, the virus can insinuate itself into human cells and replicate at a phenomenal rate. While effective medicines exist to slow it down, it is cunning and can mutate, so far surviving all attempts to annihilate it.

THE HUMAN IMMUNODEFICIENCY virus (HIV) is an infectious germ that has been described as a brain without a body. It has to hijack a cell in order to replicate and survive. It does this by entering and infecting a human host.

In a cruel twist, HIV cripples the body's immune system, the very system we need to protect ourselves against viruses and other disease agents such as bacteria and parasites. The body's immune system is comprised of, amongst other things, CD4 cells (also known as T-cells). The virus invades these cells and tricks them into making copies of itself. It does this by disguising itself in such a way as to fool the CD4 cell to let it in. It then enters the cell's brain (nucleus) by pretending to be part of the cell itself. Once in the nucleus, it integrates its own DNA into the DNA of the hijacked cell and then, when the cell makes new proteins (the bread and butter task of all cells), it inadvertently makes new viruses as well. In effect, the cell becomes an HIV factory. Literally billions of copies of the virus are created daily in the body of an infected person. The newly formed viruses leave the infected cell to invade others, staging in effect a hostile takeover of the body's entire immune system.

CD4 cells are sometimes referred to as the body's army. Initially HIV knocks off individual soldiers but the army remains strong enough to withstand the slings and arrows of life's daily contact with disease. At this stage, an infected person is said to be HIV-positive. A person who is HIV-positive looks and *is* healthy but can at this point infect others if his or her bodily fluids (most commonly sperm, vaginal fluid, breastmilk or blood) are transferred to another person.

Over time, however, the virus destroys the bulk of the army and when the CD4 count falls below a certain critical amount (less than 200 cells per microliter of blood) the body has increasing difficulty fighting off diseases and becomes susceptible to opportunistic infections (also called AIDS-defining illnesses, see

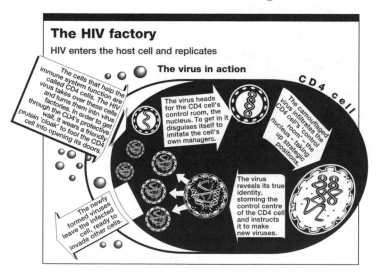

The HIV factory

HIV enters the host cell and replicates

The virus in action

CD4 cell

The cells that help the immune system function are called CD4 cells. The HIV virus takes over these cells and turns them into virus factories. In order to get through the CD4's protective wall, it wears a friendly protein 'cloak' to fool the CD4 cell into opening its doors.

The virus heads for the CD4 cell's control room, the nucleus. To get in it disguises itself to imitate the cell's own managers.

The camouflaged virus infiltrates the CD4 cell's control room – taking up strategic nucleus positions.

The virus reveals its true identity, storming the control centre of the CD4 cell and instructs it to make new viruses.

The newly formed viruses leave the infected cell, ready to invade other cells.

later in this chapter) which in the majority of cases, unless treated, will result in death. At this stage, the person is said to have AIDS. It may take anything between 5 to 15 years after infection before AIDS becomes manifest.

AIDS stands for 'Acquired Immuno Deficiency Syndrome'. The disease is 'acquired' as it is contracted from something (bodily fluid) that is not one's own. It is an 'immuno-deficiency disease' because, as described above, it attacks and undermines the body's immune system, and is called a 'syndrome' because it is comprised of a range of symptoms and diseases – called 'opportunistic infections' – that together paint the AIDS portrait.

The World Health Organization (WHO) has identi-fied four stages of HIV infection. Each stage represents a decline in the immune system character-ized by more serious and frequent opportunistic infections.[2]

Stage 1: There are usually no signs that a person is infected. Lymph glands may be swollen but essentially the person is healthy and can remain in this stage for many years.

Stage 2: With moderate immune deficiency the body becomes more prone to illness. Minor skin problems, colds and weight loss may occur during this phase. Herpes Zoster (also known as Shingles) often also occurs.

Stage 3: With an increasingly compromised immune system, more serious problems begin to occur. These include profound weight loss, chronic diarrhea, fever, oral thrush (a fungus in the mouth), vaginal thrush, pneumonia and tuberculosis (TB).

Stage 4: This stage is characterized by very serious dis-eases, some of which are seldom found in HIV-negative people. These include a lung infection known as pneu-mocystis carinii pneumonia, esophageal thrush (a fungal infection in the throat), infections of the brain such as toxoplasmosis and cryptococcal meningitis, severe diarrhea, continued profound weight loss and cancers such as Kaposi's Sarcoma.

The revenge of the Flat Earthers

There is a minority opinion of people who believe that HIV is not the cause of AIDS. However, an overwhelming body of research across the globe in countries of both the North and South, confirm that HIV causes AIDS. Internationally, the Bradford-Hill criteria (see box) are used to determine the cause of a disease. HIV meets all of these criteria.

How is HIV transmitted?

HIV lives in high concentrations in certain body fluids such as sperm, blood, vaginal secretions and breast-milk. If these fluids in an infected person come into contact with the blood of another person, this person is at risk of becoming infected with HIV.

Sex

Most people become infected during sex where the sperm or vaginal secretions containing the virus enter the bloodstream of an uninfected partner. The virus can cross through the membrane lining of the vagina, anus or inside of the penis, especially if there are tears or cuts present as this puts it in direct contact with the body's bloodstream. The presence of sexually transmitted infections (STIs) increases the risk of infection

---

The Bradford-Hill criteria

These international criteria are used to determine the cause of a disease. According to the criteria:

1 The cause must precede the disease
2 There must be a strong statistical association between the cause and the disease
3 There must be a biologically plausible explanation of how the cause results in the disease and
4 Higher doses of the cause must lead to more disease

HIV as the cause of AIDS meets all four of these criteria. ∎

because they cause sores or breaks in the mucosal lining and also increase inflammation. Inflammation increases the concentration of white blood cells close to the surface of the vagina, anus or penis. This both increases the risk of HIV uptake from an infected partner and also the risk of transmission, as in an infected person these white blood cells will contain the HIV.

Any sex which increases the likelihood of tearing is considered high risk. Anal sex is the most risky but any kind of rough sex or sex without adequate lubrication will be as dangerous. While adequate foreplay used to be a plea from women for more pleasure, it has now taken on life-preservation proportions. As noted in chapter 2, in some parts of the world 'dry' sex is considered more pleasurable for the man and many women will insert herbs and substances in their vagina to accommodate this, placing themselves at high risk of contracting HIV through abrasions. In one of the more bizarre twists, a woman's natural lubrication is in some countries believed to signify infidelity. Many women 'dry up' their vaginas to avoid the consequences which could well range from violence to abandonment.

Rape increases the risk of HIV infection as it is often physically violent and thus more likely to cause tears that bring infected sperm directly into contact with the raped person's bloodstream. Gang rape jacks up the risk even more because the chances of being exposed to an HIV-infected person are multiplied. Antiretroviral (ARV) medication, given shortly after rape, is believed to help prevent transmission. Known as 'post-exposure prophylaxis' the medication works by lowering the initial viral load and thereby preventing the virus from taking hold in the body.

Blood

Nowadays, transmission through blood takes place primarily through the sharing of needles and syringes with infected people. This is common with intravenous drug use, already widespread in Europe and North America, and increasing in countries such as Russia and other regions including Asia. Infection through direct blood to blood contact used to happen more frequently through blood transfusions when laboratories were unaware of the risks of HIV transmission. Today, most laboratories screen donated blood thoroughly for HIV but in some countries where standards are low or screening is absent, transfusions remain risky. Many people in China and India for example have become infected in this way.

Sharing of razor blades and toothbrushes are not recommended as both allow for the transmission of HIV through blood contact – razors through cut skin and toothbrushes through bleeding gums and open mouth sores.

Certain jobs place people at increased risk of infection via blood. Health-workers are an example as they may suffer needle injuries. It must be said, however, that there have not been many cases where transmission has taken place in this way because the health-worker needs to be directly exposed to a substantial amount of blood for infection to occur. Post-exposure prophylaxis, using ARVs, has been shown to prevent infection in these cases.

Newborn babies are also at risk of infection through exposure to its mother's blood during labor if the mother is infected. A pregnant woman has about a one in three (33 per cent) chance of transmitting the virus to her baby. Mother-to-child transmission (MTCT) can take place during pregnancy, labor and through breastfeeding; however 70 per cent of all such cases occur during labor and delivery. Today, with the advent of antiretroviral therapy to combat HIV/AIDS, pregnant mothers and their newborn babies can be given a course of ARVs of varying duration depending on the type or combination of ARVs used. Prolonged and extensive use of such drugs targeting the three points of transmission (during pregnancy, labor and breastfeeding) has virtually eliminated MTCT in certain countries of the North.

Shorter courses of ARV drugs such as AZT or Nevirapine (a substantially cheaper medication) during labor and delivery have been shown to reduce HIV transmission by at least half and offer hope to poor countries in providing an affordable, sustainable, simple and feasible strategy for reducing this form of HIV spread.

Breastmilk

The virus is present in large quantities in the milk of infected mothers, who may transmit the virus to their newborns through breastfeeding. About 15 per cent of all cases of HIV transmission from mother to baby take place this way. In wealthier areas this problem is bypassed by giving the baby a powdered breastmilk substitute. But as seen in chapter 2 this is not an option for mothers in poor communities with little access to clean water, since the risk of a child dying from diarrhea and dehydration caused by dirty water and bottles remains greater than the risk of passing on HIV through breastmilk. Recent research suggests that six months of uninterrupted, *exclusive* breastfeeding may be protective and has been shown to reduce transmission to about 5 to 8 per cent. Although it is unclear exactly why, it seems that if breastmilk is mixed with anything else, even water, this can cause the baby's delicate intestinal lining to tear – resulting in a higher risk of HIV-transmission through breastfeeding. In countries where antiretroviral drugs are affordable, mothers are given the option of ARV therapy in combination with exclusive breastfeeding for six months or bottle-feeding, which together greatly diminish the risk of transmission. Ultimately, all mothers should be given the information so that they can make an informed choice. While battles are fought for universal access to drugs and breastmilk substitutes, tragically, in our inequitable world this choice is limited for many poor women.

How to tell if you are HIV-positive

Because HIV can exist in the blood of an infected person for many years before it destroys the immune system, people with HIV look healthy and have no symptoms of illness. Therefore, the only way to know if you are HIV-positive is by having a test. There are a number of different types of tests which can be done using blood, urine, semen, vaginal secretions or sputum. When a person becomes infected with HIV, the body's immune system produces antibodies to fight the virus. The most common test will check for the presence of HIV antibodies in your blood.

A more expensive test is available that detects HIV directly. This test, known as the Polymerase Chain Reaction test (PCR) can also detect the amount of virus in your blood. The antibody tests are used most frequently and involve different techniques (such as the ELISA, EIA and Western Blots). Antibody tests are also able to measure whether someone has been recently infected with HIV or if a person has a long-standing infection.[3]

Rapid tests are now available that can provide a result within 15 minutes but the majority of tests take a few days to be conducted in a laboratory. All reputable laboratories will double-check any HIV-positive test results by running the sample using a different testing product. Extensive studies throughout the world show that the HIV tests are very accurate and when used together with a second test, the probability of an error is minimal.

It is important to remember though that the antibodies to the virus are not detectable in the blood in the first few weeks after infection because it takes some time for the body to develop them. This phase is known as the window period. If tested during this time, using the standard antibody detection tests, the result may be negative. Also important to consider is that children born to HIV-positive women usually have their mother's HIV antibodies in their blood even if they themselves are not infected. These antibodies can take over 18 months to clear from the baby's body and until then, a positive test cannot be taken to mean a child is HIV-positive. The PCR test however will accurately determine the child's HIV status within a few weeks of birth.

Pre- and post-test counseling are considered the right of every person undergoing an HIV test. Counseling is vital in helping a person prepare themselves for the results and in promoting protective behaviors. Informing a person with HIV of their rights is an essential component of counseling, given the global climate of discrimination and stigma for HIV-positive people.

Safe sex – does it exist?

The only kind of totally safe sex is no sex. This has led many politically-correct AIDS prevention workers to advise those 'getting some', to have 'safer sex'. While 'ABC' prevention campaigns around the world have reduced the scope of safer sex to encompass Abstinence, Be faithful or wear a Condom, safer sex can thankfully involve more creative measures. Sex shops and clubs throughout the world have developed erotized ways of having safer sex and after years on the fringes condoms, latex surgical gloves, dental dams and plastic wrap for oral sex have become more acceptable accoutrements. Sex toys are also good, but if shared, are best used with a condom. Condom use in the porn industry is becoming more common although 'come' shots still seem to demand endless visuals of free-flying sperm.

Abstinence is recommended for the very young and those who are willing and able to make this lifestyle choice. Transmission risk is zero. For those who can't or don't want to make this choice there are many other options.

Being faithful is only safe if both you and your partner have already been tested for HIV and are both negative. Obviously the window period must be taken into account. If you then remain monogamous, unprotected sex is totally safe. Unfortunately, the ABC message has misled many people who engage in 'serial monogamy' to be lulled into a sense of false security because they are 'faithful' to their current partner.

Safer sex means making sure you don't come into direct contact with your partner's blood, semen, vaginal fluids or breastmilk. It also means protecting your partner from yours. In the past, traditional societies had innovative ways of engaging in safe sex as a means of preventing pregnancy. In parts of Africa, for example, young boys were instructed in the art of thigh sex (rubbing their penis between a girl's thighs) as part of their initiation into manhood. Some AIDS prevention programs have encouraged the revival of such practices. Women in general have long advocated more imaginative and varied forms of sex than just penetration. In that respect, perhaps things are looking up for them as people are compelled to get more experimental. Massage, more focus on the clitoris and

Get it on

Billions of dollars have been spent on the promotion and distribution of condoms since the AIDS epidemic began but it is worth going through the basics of their use again here. Lubricated latex condoms should be used whenever a person engages in anal or vaginal sex. Latex is recommended because lambskin condoms don't block HIV or other sexually-transmitted infections and because polyurethane condoms tend to break more easily. Lubricant keeps things smooth but is only safe if it is water-based lubricant as oil will weaken the latex, making the condom more likely to break. Make sure the condom expiration date has not passed. Condoms are only safe if properly used. This includes ensuring the penis is hard before putting a condom on, ensuring the condom is correctly applied – rolled down all the way with a tip at the top to leave space for the sperm and to ensure there are no air bubbles which can also cause the condom to break. And of course condoms should only be used once and then thrown away. Don't get them punctured, don't keep in places where they can get too hot or damaged, like in direct sunlight, in a car's glove compartment or in a wallet. ■

G-spot, mutual masturbation and a greater interest in kissing may result in a great many more orgasms for women. Having said that, men seem unlikely to forgo their joys of penetration and so on the menu of safe sex, condoms remain the main course (see box p 77).

The word on oral sex

Opinion is still divided on the safety of oral sex. Some people see it as extremely low risk while others believe that it should never be tried without a condom or dental dam. It is certainly less risky than anal or vaginal sex because the mucous membrane lining the mouth is much tougher, thicker and more resilient than that of the vagina or anus, so it is more difficult for HIV to break through.

Certainly, blow jobs are safest if you use a condom. Giving a blow job is more risky than getting one. This is because there is more chance that HIV-infected fluid will enter the body, especially if there are cuts or bleeding gums in the mouth. Oral-vaginal sex is low risk relative to oral-penis sex, although the likelihood of infection increases when there is menstrual blood or an unusual vaginal discharge. Dental dams or plastic wraps make this form of pleasure even safer.

Precum – the small amount of fluid emitted prior to ejaculation – contains less HIV than semen and therefore exposure to precum is less risky. However, while the risk has been described as minimal under normal circumstances (that is, in the absence of sores, cuts or tears in the mouth or genitals), it is not risk-free – so better to use a condom. Firstly, without one you will still be exposed to sexually transmitted infections (STIs) which in turn increase the risk of contracting HIV. Secondly, contrary to popular belief, precum can definitely lead to pregnancy.

Kissing is considered safe as HIV, although present in saliva, is found in such small quantities so as to make the risk of transmission negligible. There is also scientific evidence that enzymes in the saliva help neutralize the virus. Deep kissing if there are open sores, small cuts on the mouth or bleeding gums should be avoided as this blood may contain sufficient infected white blood cells to transmit HIV.

'Opportunistic' infections[4]

Opportunistic infections are those that move in on a person's compromised immune system. Many of them are only found in people with HIV. Others, like tuberculosis (TB), are more serious if they occur in someone with HIV as the immune system of an HIV-negative person has more chance of fighting them off.

TB is the most common life-threatening opportunistic infection for HIV-positive people in Africa. The TB epidemic was already out of control in many parts of the world but is now exploding exponentially as a result of the AIDS epidemic. The epidemics are mutually reinforcing. The TB bacillus is spread easily from one person to another through coughing, sneezing or breathing. Poverty, with its concomitant overcrowded living conditions and poor nutrition, provides the perfect environment for the spread of TB. While all people with HIV are at greater risk of contracting TB, the mix of poverty and HIV is the reason that TB is the most common cause of death among people with AIDS in many parts of Africa. While TB can be cured, its treatment requires strict compliance to a multiple drug regimen for a period of at least 6 months.

Candidiasis is another common opportunistic infection associated with AIDS. Colloquially known as 'thrush', it is usually a harmless but intensely irritating fungal infection for the many women who regularly fall prey to its vaginal form. A short course of antifungal treatment will usually banish it. In an immune-compromised person with AIDS however, thrush becomes florid and can affect the mucous membranes of the mouth, vagina, esophagus and skin. It is particularly dangerous in its oral-esophageal forms as it prevents a person from eating, undermining the nutritional status necessary to keep the immune system strong.

There are medications available to treat thrush but as with many AIDS-related drugs, battles have been waged to make them affordable to all, regardless of a person's or their country's bank balance.

Until recently US pharmaceutical giant Pfizer held the patent to its anti-fungal drug Diflucan and charged anything between $8 and $28 for the pill. Pfizer's sales to wealthy US and European patients are worth $1 billion a year. Thailand can produce a generic Diflucan for less than 30 cents. But for many years Pfizer refused to provide the drug cheaply to developing countries or to allow countries to manufacture their own cheaper generics. Thankfully, with the patent now expired on Diflucan, cheaper generic forms of this drug may now be made more widely available. There is more about this in the next chapter.

Other common opportunistic infections in AIDS are gasteroenteritic infections causing chronic diarrhea, cryptococcal meningitis (a fungal infection of the membranes lining the brain) and pneumocystis carinii pneumonia (PCP) a previously rare kind of lung infection.

Treatment is available for most opportunistic infections, although in advanced AIDS the medication may become ineffective. Antiretroviral therapy can reverse HIV's damage to the immune system and can lessen the likelihood as well as the severity of opportunistic infections.

Living positively with 'Aunty Aida'

Gay South African lingo refers to the virus as 'Aunty Aida' – reflecting as it were a strange truce with an unwelcome relative. In the early days of the epidemic, people conflated being HIV-positive with having AIDS. Lack of access to adequate counseling and support drove many people to suicide, believing death was imminent. Nowadays, recognizing that someone can live many healthy years before becoming sick with AIDS, and given that life-prolonging drugs are now available – at least for those who can afford them – people have found ways to live positively with the virus.

Living a healthy life

Eating well, exercising regularly and getting plenty of rest all help to keep one's immune system fortified. Avoiding smoking and alcohol are also essential. This will go a long way to keeping one's body healthy and staving off AIDS.

While many people erroneously believe they are at risk from a person with HIV through casual contact, the truth is that it is the person living with HIV who is more vulnerable to getting infections from others. Avoiding infections and treating opportunistic ones as soon as possible will also help to protect one's body.

The prevention and treatment of opportunistic infections during Stages 1 and 2 of HIV (see p 70) is essential to enhance the quality of one's life as well as to prolong it.

Antiretroviral drugs

The discovery of antiretroviral (ARV) drugs has changed the course of the epidemic in countries of the North. Unconscionably, these medications are out of the price range of most countries in the South with the result that millions of people are dying of a disease that has largely become a manageable, chronic illness in richer parts of the world.

ARVs cannot cure AIDS but they can prevent HIV from reproducing inside the body, giving the immune system a chance to recover and fight back. This can lower the viral load (amount of virus in the body) substantially. There are 14 different kinds of ARVs but many more are being researched.

The three main types are firstly Nucleoside Reverse Transcriptase Inhibitors (affectionately known as

'Nukes'). These act by mimicking the natural building blocks of the virus's DNA. They are 'wrongly' incorporated into growing viral DNA and abort their replication. AZT and 3TC, commonly used ARVs, are both Nukes.

Then you get 'Non-Nukes' which are Non-Nucleoside Reverse Transcriptase Inhibitors. They work by blocking a part of the enzyme necessary for the production of the viral DNA. This stops HIV from being formed.

The third category is the Protease Inhibitors which work by preventing the maturation of viral particles after viral proteins have formed.

There is overwhelming evidence that ARVs work for the prevention of mother-to-child transmission and the treatment of people with AIDS. For the latter, a cocktail of at least three drugs is recommended. Known as triple therapy, combination therapy or HAART (Highly Active Antiretroviral Therapy), studies have shown an improvement of over 70 per cent in the reduction of illness and death in people taking these drugs, compared to those not on treatment.[5,6] There is more on HAART in chapter 4.

ARVs are taken for the following:

1 To reduce the risk of mother-to-child transmission (MTCT).

2 As prophylaxis for people exposed to HIV through occupational injuries such as health-workers, or through rape. This is known as Post-Exposure Prophylaxis or PEP.

3 To treat people who are infected with HIV so that they can live healthier and longer lives. Used in combination therapy the drugs work together to tackle HIV from different angles. Only once a person's CD4 count has dropped to a certain level (usually under 200 per microliter of blood), or in the presence of AIDS-defining illnesses, does a person with HIV need to go onto HAART. The medication must be taken every day for life although many doctors are

now recommending intermittent periods of 'drug holidays'.

Some countries, reluctant to embark on major treatment programs, argue that HAART can have serious side-effects which militate against their use. However, this is the case with most drugs, including common headache tablets. Chemotherapy often has far more serious side-effects than HAART yet chemotherapy's use as a cancer treatment is not questioned. When one considers that for people with cancer or AIDS the alternative is usually death, the drug benefits far outweigh their risks. People on HAART are monitored for side-effects and when serious, alternative combinations of drugs are recommended.[7]

As with all infections, drug resistance is also a major challenge. Resistance occurs when the organism gets wise to medication and outsmarts it by mutating. This happens with extended or incorrect use and the resistant virus begins to destroy the immune system again. Such patients can change to a different set of drugs although eventually they may run out of alternatives. But in most people taking their drugs correctly this only occurs after many years by which time new medications may well be available. Of great concern though is the transmission of resistant strains to other people, thereby limiting their treatment options too

---

Steve's story

Steve Mueller in Toronto, Canada, is a warm, articulate 42-year-old with sharp sculpted features, a halo of black curls and a hacking cough – the legacy of a battle with HIV which is not yet over. When he got sick in the early 1990s his world was shattered. He lost his job and his partner who was also HIV-positive died within a year. Steve then contracted meningitis, one of the 'opportunistic infections'.

'The doctors told me in June 1995 that I was unlikely to see Christmas. I'd gone from 180 to 120 pounds and I was still losing weight. Then I started on the AIDS cocktail; it literally pulled me back from the edge. They called guys like me, who were dying and then bounced back, the Lazarus men'. ∎

New Internationalist No 346, June 2002. www.newint.org

---

and making the epidemic harder to control. Again, this is not a legitimate reason to withhold treatment: for example, despite resistance to some drugs, TB patients continue to be treated. Without ARV, people will die of AIDS irrespective of whether or not they have a resistant strain of HIV.

Patients on HAART must undergo regular monitoring. This includes CD4 counts which measure the strength of the immune system as well as various blood tests to identify side-effects. These tests are expensive and, along with the price of ARVs themselves, are a focus of struggle for AIDS activists too.

An AIDS vaccine – medicine's Holy Grail

Despite initial hopes, a vaccine for AIDS is unfortunately still many years off. The big challenge facing vaccine development is that the virus mutates rapidly, thereby outwitting vaccines designed to stave off its original form. Also there are many different strains of HIV in circulation so it is not clear if it will be possible for one vaccine to work against all variants.

Traditionally, vaccines are made by using a killed or weakened form of the virus itself, which stimulates the immune system to produce antibodies before the real thing comes its way. Scientists are currently researching the use of harmless bits of HIV to ensure that vaccination cannot cause a person to become infected.

Vaccines can take ages to develop. First you have to do your homework in the laboratory. Then they are tested on animals (a contentious issue for some people) and only then do you venture into human trials. Tim Tucker, Director of the South African AIDS Vaccine Initiative (SAAVI) puts it in perspective: 'We are not running a short race here. We are running a marathon – probably an ultra marathon.'[8]

Much of the research has been criticized for focusing only on the viral strains that are common in the North – where the money is – while neglecting strains more common to countries in South. However, more recently, major vaccine research initiatives have begun in countries such as Brazil, Cuba, South Africa and India.

Vaccine development is a minefield of ethical dilemmas and concerns. Who goes onto the trials, what are the benefits and ultimately who really benefits, what are the risks to participants? These are some of the tricky areas researchers must navigate. The rights of those involved, including genuine, informed consent to participate should be paramount.

Remarkably soon after HIV was first discovered, the US Congress' Office of Technology brought out a review of the Public Health Service's response. The report stated: 'We hope to have a vaccine [against HIV] ready for testing in about two years' and ironically concluded with 'yet another terrible disease is about to yield to patience, persistence and outright genius.'[9] That was in the mid-1980s. Almost 20 years later, estimates are that we are probably more than a decade away from the elusive vaccine. While a vaccine is no panacea – programs aimed at the prevention, care and treatment of HIV and AIDS will remain part of life for years to come – it will make a huge impact on the magnitude of the epidemic. Meantime, though, you'd be well advised to keep your condoms.

1 Interview with Musa Njoko by D Renzon, *Elle,* October 2002, p 44. **2** Cited in 'AIDS: Know the Facts', published by Soul City Institute for Health and Development Communication, The Health Systems Trust, University of Natal 2002. **3** 'AIDS: Know the Facts', op. cit. **4** 'AIDS: Know the Facts', op. cit. **5** Pallala et al, *New England Journal of Medicine* 1998, 338 (13): 853-60. **6** Mocroft et al, 'Changing Patterns of Mortality Across Europe in Patients Infected with HIV-1', *Lancet,* 352, 1725-30, 1998. **7** 'AIDS: Know the Facts', published by Soul City Institute for Health and Development Communication, The Health Systems Trust, University of Natal 2002. **8** Interview with Tim Tucker by M Rotchford Galloway, 'Coordinating the SAAVI Family', in *MRC AIDS Bulletin*, Vol 11, No 2, July 2002. **9** 'Review of the Public Health Service's Response to AIDS', Washington, DC: US Congress, Office of Technology Assessment, February, p 29, cited on www.avert.org/his81_86.htm

4 The politics of profit

'We wonder what is deadlier in sub-Saharan Africa – AIDS or businessmen with briefcases full of patent applications.'
Christopher Ouma, Kenyan doctor, Action Aid.[1]

'Nearly 34 million people in our world are at this moment dying [of AIDS, in 2000]. And they are dying because they don't have the privilege that I have, of purchasing my health and life... Now why should I have the privilege...when 34 million people in the resource poor world are falling ill, feeling sick to death, and are dying? That to me...seems a moral inequity of such fundamental proportions that no one can look at it and fail to be spurred to thought and action about it. That is something which we in Africa cannot accept. It is something that the developed world also cannot accept.'
Edwin Cameron, Constitutional Court judge who is HIV-positive, South Africa.

The advent of antiretroviral (ARV*) therapy for the treatment of HIV/AIDS has changed the nature of the pandemic in many parts of the world. HIV/AIDS has become a manageable, chronic disease in countries that can afford these life-saving drugs. But the majority of people cannot access them because of profiteering by the pharmaceutical industry, backed by trade agreements forged in the interests of wealthy nations.

IN THE MID-1980s it was hard to find space in San Francisco's *Bay Area Reporter* obituary columns, so many people were dying in their prime of AIDS. Things got so bad that newspaper employed a full-time 'obituary' editor. Then something remarkable happened. Highly

---

* ARVs are also used to prevent mother-to-child transmission (MTCT) of HIV. Programs for the prevention of MTCT, which include the provision of antiretroviral medication, have practically wiped out the pediatric AIDS epidemic in Europe and North America.

Active Antiretroviral Therapy (HAART) was introduced in 1996 and the number of people dying from AIDS began to drop dramatically. In August 1998 the obituary editor was retrenched and the newspaper ran a banner headline which read: 'No Obits!! Death Takes A Holiday'.[2]

In just a few years, HAART has transformed HIV/AIDS from a fatal illness into a manageable disease. As with diabetes, hypertension and other chronic, incurable diseases, a combination of lifestyle changes and ARV medication can successfully extend both the quality and the quantity of life for HIV-positive people.

While HAART is commonly thought of as purely a treatment response, its role in prevention is also increasingly recognized. Firstly, it prevents the onset of opportunistic infections (see chapter 3). Secondly, with something life-saving to offer people, more come voluntarily to be tested, counseled and helped. By bringing people into counseling, which has shown to improve safe-sex behavior, further infections can be prevented.

Conversely, there is very little incentive for voluntary testing if there is no treatment after diagnosis. After all, what's in it for people; why should they bother? De-linking AIDS from death also helps to overcome the tremendous obstacle presented by the stigma associated with the epidemic, undoubtedly one of the greatest barriers we face in dealing with HIV/AIDS. As with cancer, stigma and denial are the offspring of the fear associated with something terminal. The 'Big C' – for an illness whose full name could not be mentioned – has become the 'Big A'. HAART presents an opportunity to reduce the stigma of HIV/AIDS allowing it to be perceived as a chronic disease which does not have to carry a death sentence.

The question of whether HAART works is no longer up for debate. As seen in the last chapter, years of sound research indicates that a cocktail of at least three ARVs, taken every day for life, *is* effective in slowing down the development of AIDS, keeping people both healthier and alive longer.

Yet despite this obvious life-saving intervention the fact remains that of the 28 million people then living with HIV/AIDS (PWAs) in sub-Saharan Africa, only about 30,000 were estimated to have benefited from ARVs by the end of 2001.[3] In Kenya, for example, 25 per cent of people are HIV-positive but only 2 per cent can afford treatment. In South Africa only a fraction of those in need are accessing triple therapy. Patent prices are unaffordable to most, costing anything from $1,200 to $2,500 (or more) a year. In some countries the annual cost of patented HAART is as much as $10,000 to $15,000. Even if Zambia were to spend its entire national income on HIV/AIDS drugs, it still could not afford to treat every person infected with HIV in the country at these prices. Thus HAART seems to further widen the ever-increasing gap between the global rich and poor.

Four issues are consistently raised to explain why HAART is not more extensively utilized: drug toxicity, drug resistance, lack of health-service infrastructure and cost.

The first three considerations are all important but surmountable and are not valid reasons for not implementing treatment programs. These issues are discussed in some detail in other chapters. But the issue at the heart of the matter is affordability.

Big Pharma – big profits

Father D'Agnostino, founder of the Nymbani children's home in Nairobi, Kenya, is justifiably angry. Declaring himself 'sick and tired of doing funerals' of the orphaned children he takes care of – children whose parents have died of AIDS and many of whom are now dying themselves – Father D'Agnostino recently announced his intention to defy Big Pharma (the pharmaceutical industry collectively) and import cheaper generic drugs from India. According to Father D'Agnostino: 'It really is the darkest side of capitalism. Pharmaceutical companies are holding the people of sub-Saharan Africa to ransom. People are dying because the cost of drugs cannot be reduced.'[4]

The simple truth is that the astronomically high cost of ARVs prevents most PWAs from receiving drugs, sentencing them to premature death. It must be one of the most pressing moral issues of our time that even today the right to be alive is still largely determined by one's ability to pay for it. Despite a plethora of international conventions enshrining the human rights of life and dignity, it seems that the intellectual property rights and the right of transnational pharmaceutical

The proof is in the pudding

Drug companies spend twice as much on marketing, advertising and administration than they do on research and development (R & D). In most cases, company profits far exceed R & D costs.

Financials for US corporations marketing top 50 drugs for older people/seniors

Company	Revenue (Net Sales in millions of dollars)	Percentage of Revenue Allocated to Profit (Net income)	Percentage of Revenue Allocated to Marketing, advertising, admin	Percentage of Revenue Allocated to R&D
Merck & Co., Inc	40,363	17%	15%	6%
Pfizer Inc.	29,574	13%	39%	15%
Bristol-Myers Squibb Co.	18,216	26%	30%	15%
Pharmacia Corporation	18,144	4%	37%	15%
Abbott Laboratories	13,746	20%	21%	10%
American Home Products Corporation	13,263	-18%	38%	13%
Eli Lilly & Co.	10,862	28%	30%	19%
Schering-Plough Corporation	9,815	25%	36%	14%
Allergan, Inc.	1,563	14%	42%	13%

corporations to make exorbitant profits rank higher. Angry activists are demanding that in the formulation and implementation of drug trade policies, public health and human rights concerns take precedence over commercial and other economic interests. This position has been endorsed by the UN, most notably in its International Guidelines on HIV/AIDS and Human Rights in July 2002. As noted in chapter 1, recent updating recognizes access to medication as essential to the attainment of the right to health (Guideline Six).

Big Pharma maintains its market monopoly through patents which prevent the production of cheaper generic drugs for at least 20 years. For many drugs, generic production would reduce the price by anything between 70-95 per cent, depending on the manufacturing costs. The industry argues that the astronomical prices of ARVs are necessary to recoup research and development (R & D) costs. Many corporations have begun to refer to themselves as 'research-based pharmaceutical companies' in an attempt to focus attention on this supposedly central aspect of their work.

Jeff Truit, an official of PhRMA (Pharmaceutical Research and Manufacturers' Association, the US pharmaceutical industry group) claims that the average drug costs $300 to $500 million to develop[5]. The industry also makes much of intellectual property rights that must be protected in the form of patents, which Abraham Lincoln claimed 'provide the fuel for the fire of genius'.

But not everyone agrees that ARVs cost the pharmaceutical companies *hundreds* of millions of dollars' worth of R & D. Activists also hotly contest the notion of 'intellectual property rights' presented by industry. They maintain that the scientific discoveries, from which the industry benefits, are the fruit of the labor of scientists and technicians which is part of a historical process of accumulation of collective knowledge.

According to James Love, director of the Consumer Project on Technology, industry claims on R & D are extremely tenuous: 'In 1997 prices, the average out-of-pocket costs of clinical trials needed for FDA [US Food and Drug Administration] approval were $25 million. Adjusted for risk, the 'per approval' cost of clinical trials was $56 million. [Higher estimates] adjust these costs somewhat higher to include 'capital costs' for financing trials, but also and most importantly the cost of preclinical research, which accounts for 70-80 per cent of the total cost of drug development in some studies. Moreover, it is often governments rather than the drug companies that pay for clinical and preclinical research.'[6]

Who really pays?

The truth is that many ARVs such as azidothymidine (AZT) were developed at the US taxpayers' expense with funding from the National Institutes of Health (NIH). It is estimated that the US Government funds 38 per cent of health care research while 10 per cent is funded by other government agencies and non-profit organizations. Thus, the private sector only funds about just over half of the total health care research, but reaps most of the profits.[7] In addition, most companies recover their R & D costs within five years of a product being patented.

According to Public Citizen, a non-profit consumer advocacy organization in Washington DC, actual spending by the pharmaceutical industry on R & D of new drugs is only about one fifth of what it says it spends. While the industry also argues that it needs to make huge profits on one drug to finance the R & D of others, Public Citizen found that: 'At most, about 22 per cent of the new drugs brought to market in the past two decades were innovative drugs that represented important therapeutic advances. Most new drugs were copycat ones that have little or no therapeutic gain over existing drugs.' Adding insult to injury, only one-tenth of pharmaceutical companies' R & D expenditure goes into drugs that account for 90 per cent of global diseases. In contrast, most of such costs are on rich world ailments such as obesity, anti-ageing treatment and chemical dependency.[8] Roy Vagelos, the former head of Merck, which controls 10 per cent of the world's pharmaceutical market, does not mince his words: 'A corporation with stockholders can't stick up a laboratory that will focus on Third World diseases because it would go broke.'[9]

Most AIDS activists recognize that the pharmaceutical industry is entitled to make profits. What is being contested, according to Zackie Achmat of South Africa's Treatment Action Campaign (TAC), is the right of the industry to 'profiteer' – to make unconscionable profits on essential, lifesaving medicines. Achmat's actions speak louder than words. The HIV-positive activist refused to take ARVs himself until the

Fat cats

Extravagant compensation packages of drug company top executives swallow up millions of dollars. This greed, rather than high research and development costs, contributes to the high cost of drugs.

The five highest-paid drug company executives – annual compensation exclusive of unexercised stock options, 2000

Executive	Company	Compensation ($ million)
William C Steere, Jr (Chairperson)	Pfizer Inc.	
John R Stafford (Chairperson & CEO)	American Home Products Corp.	
Edward M Scolnick (Executive VP)	Merck & Co, Inc.	
Richard Jay Cogan	Schering-Plough Corporation	
David W Anstice (President, the Americas)	Merck & Co, Inc.	

South African Government took steps to make the drugs accessible to all.

So just how much profits are the drug companies fighting to protect? Profits that are undreamed of in any other industry. the combined worth of the top five pharmaceutical companies is twice the combined GDP of all the sub-Saharan African countries. According to *USA Today*, sales of ARVs alone total roughly $3 billion a year.[10] In 2000, the pharmaceutical industry was the most profitable US industry with margins nearly four times the average of *Fortune* magazine's top 500 companies. In 2001 the industry topped all three of *Fortune*'s measures of profitability – the third decade in which the industry has been at or near the top.

Families USA is a non-profit consumer health organization. According to its executive director, Ron Pollack: 'High prices are… associated with record-breaking profits and enormous compensation for top drug company executives. If meaningful steps are taken to ameliorate fast-growing drug prices, it is corporate profits, expenditures on marketing and high executive compensation that are more likely to be affected, not research and development.'[11]

Despite these massive profits, pharmaceutical companies pay less in taxes than any other US industry. According to the Congressional Research Service (CRS), the drug industry pays a rate of 16.2 per cent relative to the industry average of 23.7 per cent. The same report states that from 1994 to 1998, the industry's profits after tax, as a percentage of sales, averaged 17 per cent which is more than three times the average rate of 5 per cent for all industries.[12] According to the CRS report the drug industry benefits more than most industries from R & D tax credits as well as foreign tax credit from sales to other countries.

The politics of patents

The pharmaceutical industry maintains its market monopoly and protects its exorbitant profits through patents which prevent the production of cheaper generic drugs for at least 20 years. The production of generic (non-patented/brand-name) drugs would greatly enhance access to ARVs for millions of people. Importing generics from countries such as India could reduce the cost of triple therapy to less than $300 per year (from $10-15,000 in the US), while Thailand believes it can reduce the price to around $200 per year.

Patents are not only placing antiretroviral drugs beyond the price range of most of the world's AIDS patients. As noted in the previous chapter, they also make unaffordable the medicines used to treat opportunistic infections associated with AIDS. For example, in Thailand, around a fifth of people with AIDS suffer from cryptococcal meningitis, an infection of the membranes that line the brain. If they remain untreated they will die a painful death in less than a month. A medicine called fluconazole, commonly prescribed for vaginal thrush, also treats esophageal candidiasis, a fungal throat infection that makes it impossible to swallow, undermining essential nutrition. The price of a patented pill of fluconazole (called Diflucan) in Thailand is $5. But Thailand can produce a generic version, called Biozole, for less than $0.28. Until 2002, Pfizer held the patent on fluconazole with sales to wealthy US and European patients worth $1 billion a year. Still it refused to provide the drug cheaply to countries of the South or to allow countries bound by intellectual property agreements to manufacture their own cheaper generics.

South African activist Zackie Achmat made a daredevil trip to Thailand to purchase Biozole and 'smuggled' the drugs back into South Africa. At the time, the drug was only available on Pfizer's patent, at greatly inflated prices ($4 compared with the generic cost of less than $0.28). As a result of Achmat's actions and the activism surrounding this, Pfizer now donates fluconazole through the South African public health system. However, these drugs are not freely available for all kinds of fungal infections. In the light of these restrictions, and the fact that donations in general are dependent on the 'goodwill' of the pharmaceutical company concerned, generic competition remains the most effective mechanism to ensure universal access.

TRIPS and trade

Drug patents are enforced internationally through the World Trade Organization (WTO) agreement known as TRIPS (Trade Related Aspects of Intellectual Property Rights). TRIPS lays out a set of minimum standards to which intellectual property law of the member states of the WTO must conform. These minimum standards make it difficult for countries to bypass Big Pharma patents and import or produce their own cheaper generics.

TRIPS does however have 'flexibility clauses' allowing member states to depart from these minimum standards, such as by allowing for the issuing of compulsory licenses for the importation or local production of cheaper generic versions of patented drugs. The licenses are said to be 'compulsory' because they don't require the permission of the patent holder. Under TRIPS, compulsory licenses include compensation for the patent holder (typically a 3-5 per cent royalty fee). Countries are free to determine the grounds on which such licenses may be issued. In the event of a national health emergency, however, TRIPS allows for compulsory licenses to be issued without certain procedural requirements being followed, such as prior negotiations with the patent holder. This makes it easier and quicker to issue licenses in such circumstances.

TRIPS' obfuscating language (which many believe is intentional) has created great confusion and allowed transnational drug companies and countries such as the US to 'bully' countries in the South by alleging they are violating TRIPS, even when they are not. It was only at the 2001 WTO ministerial conference in Doha, Qatar (and more recently in 2002) that an attempt was made to clarify for the world exactly what TRIPS' public health 'safeguards' entail. In an important declaration the ministers announced that they recognized the tremendous 'gravity of the public health problems afflicting many developing and least developed countries', naming the AIDS epidemic as one of these. While the Doha Declaration on the TRIPS Agreement and Public Health recognized 'that intellectual property protection is important for the development of new medicines' it also acknowledged the concerns about the effect this has on prices.

Importantly, the Doha Declaration states that 'the TRIPS agreement does not and should not prevent members from taking measures to protect public health. Accordingly, while reiterating our commitment to the TRIPS agreement, we affirm that the Agreement can and should be interpreted and implemented in a manner supportive of WTO members' right to protect public health, and in particular, to promote access to medicines for all. In this connection, we reaffirm the right of WTO members to use to the full the provisions in the TRIPS Agreement which provide flexibility for this purpose.' It states that these flexibilities include 'each member's right to determine what constitutes "a national emergency or other circumstances of extreme urgency"' and that public health crises, including those relating to HIV/AIDS, can represent such circumstances. This was a very significant development as countries would no longer have to rely on the WTO to determine if they were indeed experiencing an emergency. 'Least developed member countries' were given until 1 January 2016 to modify their national legislation to comply with the TRIPS agreement.

The US and Switzerland, home to many transnational drug companies, tried unsuccessfully to block the Doha Declaration, proposing a weaker version.

They have also used subsequent TRIPS discussions to undermine it and to impede further movement on one important question left unanswered by the Doha discussions. The question is 'how are poorer countries that cannot afford to manufacture their own generic drugs going to access cheap drugs?' given the shrinking pool of exporting countries.

The pool is shrinking because as generic-producing countries such as India and Brazil become TRIPS-compliant, their ability to sell abroad is curtailed. This is because TRIPS limits the amount of drugs a company can produce for export under a compulsory license. Also, fewer countries able to produce generics are willing or able to withstand the pressure from the North and the transnational pharmaceutical industry not to issue compulsory licenses allowing for exportation. So even if a poor country issues its own compulsory license, it will not be that easy to import generic drugs. Thanks to the obstructions, a stalemate was reached on this issue and the debate continues.

One rule for the rich...

Ironically, when faced with the post-September 11 anthrax scare, the very same US government that threatened countries with sanctions if they disregarded patent laws on antiretrovirals declared it would disregard the Bayer AG patent on the anthrax antibiotic Cipro. According to a *New York Times* editorial in October 2001 when the Government wanted to stockpile Cipro, Health and Human Services Secretary Tommy Thompson persuaded Bayer, the patent holder, to cut the price of the drug by threatening to buy generic versions. Anthrax, the article went on, had killed a handful of Americans at the time. Arguably millions were at risk. AIDS however has already killed 22 million people globally and stands to kill millions more.

The US double standard on compulsory licensing is even more widespread. Its government stated before the Geneva conference in 1999 that it does not support the compulsory licensing of patents, regarding them as unnecessary. Yet according to the meeting's report, the US has 'liberally applied this tool in its own domestic market in hundreds of cases. Licenses on patents have been granted in diverse fields including biotechnology, pharmaceuticals, aerospace, military technology, air pollution, computers and nuclear energy. The US has traditionally used compulsory licenses to counteract anti-competitive practices and a significant number have been granted royalty-free. In addition, many have been authorized for non-commercial government use.'[13] According to the *New York Times* report, an outraged Professor Krisantha Weerasuriya of Sri Lanka's University of Colombo complained bitterly that 'as a public health worker in the developing world, I feel like a child being told by the developed world to "do as we say and not as we do"'.

Another device for accessing drugs at a lower price is parallel importation. This means that a patented medicine can be bought from the same producer in another country, usually at a lower price. This is possible as drug companies sell their medicines at different prices in different countries. TRIPS allows countries to determine their own laws regarding parallel importation and as a result, this is a common practice in Europe. However, poorer countries face the same pressures preventing them from using this avenue as they do with compulsory licensing.

Corporate bullying

AIDS and other diseases are big business and in reality, TRIPS was drawn up by rich countries to protect their business interests. As the world's most profitable industry, Big Pharma's financial muscle buys it considerable political leverage: it spent $75 million a year and more than $256 million over a 5-year period to lobby US legislators. Alarmingly, there is one pharmaceutical industry lobbyist for every two members of Congress. During the 2000 US presidential elections, an unprecedented $24.4 million was spent by Big Pharma, 70 per cent going to the Republican Party.[14] It is this political clout that led to the TRIPS Agreement being passed in the first place. Before TRIPS countries were free to produce generics without the yards of red tape. Few poor countries had intellectual property laws and Brazil and Thailand for example were able to develop thriving generic drug industries. These countries must now align their domestic law with TRIPS as a condition of membership within the WTO.

Hefty political contributions continue to pay off, with the US using all available means to close TRIPS' 'flexibility clauses' and lobbying for tougher rules protecting intellectual property rights at world forums. In 1995, the Clinton administration sided with the pharmaceutical companies by repealing a law requiring products developed in part due to research at National Institutes of Health laboratories to be 'reasonably priced'. The US also continues to intimidate countries wanting to produce generics. For example,

Big spenders

The pharmaceutical industry makes weighty contributions to political parties.

Top 10 soft money, political action committees (PAC) and individual pharmaceutical company campaign contributors in the US, 1997-1998

Company	Amount	Democrats	Republicans
Pfizer Inc.	$1,103,180	$210,850	$892,330
Bristol-Myers Squibb Co.	$827,324	$216,650	$610,674
Eli Lilly & Co.	$712,173	$205,824	$505,849
Glaxo Wellcome Inc.	$687,751	$146,825	$539,726
Novartis Corp	$638,592	$179,250	$459,342
Schering-Plough Corporation	$486,919	$109,362	$377,557
Rhone-Poulenc Inc.	$467,575	$169,500	$298,075
Merck & Co., Inc.	$351,228	$93,496	$257,732
Abbott Laboratories	$312,971	$56,672	$256,049
American Home Products Corporation	$301,225	$75,439	$225,261

Data from the FEC, 4/1/99. Totals include contributions from subsidiaries. Lobbying data based on documents filed with the Secretary of State's office, 5/11/99, from Bailey, H, 'Bitter Pills: the battle over prescription drug prices', Center for Responsive Politics Money in Politics Alert, 5 (17), 17 May 1999. (Cited in P Bond, 'Globalization, Pharmaceutical Pricing and South African Health Policy: Managing Confrontation with US Firms and Politicians', International Journal of Health Services, Vol 29, No 4, 1999.)

it threatened to withdraw a special deal to the Dominican Republic for the export of textiles unless the country scrapped plans for compulsory licensing and parallel importing. Brazil and India have also been threatened with American sanctions.[15] Thailand was forced to drop its plan to manufacture the anti-retroviral ddI after the US threatened trade sanctions on some of Thailand's key exports. ddI is exclusively marketed by Bristol-Myers Squibb, although the US Government played a significant role in the invention of the drug itself.

In what the non-governmental organization Oxfam refers to as 'corporate bullying', transnational drug companies have used threats and legal action to try to stop the efforts of countries such as South Africa, Brazil and Thailand to produce cheap medicines. Glaxo Wellcome (now GlaxoSmithKline) threatened legal action against the Indian generics company Cipla for trying to provide Ghana and Uganda with a cheap version of Combivir – a pill which combines AZT and 3TC, of which at least AZT was developed in large part with US taxpayers' money.

South Africa stands its ground

South Africa was also threatened with trade sanctions if it did not alter certain clauses in proposed legislation, particularly section 15C in the 1997 Medicines and Related Substances Control Amendment Act (Medicines Act) which would allow for, amongst other things, parallel importation. Attempts to pressure South Africa to change this clause failed. As a result, the Pharmaceutical Manufacturers' Association, on behalf of 39 international pharmaceutical firms, took the South African Government to court to prevent the Act from being promulgated, claiming it was unconstitutional and a violation of TRIPS. This was despite the fact that TRIPS allows states to determine their own rules regarding parallel imports, without fear of WTO disputes. While the companies maintained the proposed legislation was in breach of their patent rights, the South African Government said the Act would allow it to improve access to and affordability of medicines through a range of different mechanisms.

Putting the squeeze on South Africa

Pressure on South Africa came from the presidents of France, Germany and Switzerland raising the issue privately with the then Deputy President, Thabo Mbeki. The US Government took the lead. In 1998, its trade representative, endorsed by the Department of State, designated South Africa as a Special 301 'Watch List' country in its annual worldwide review of intellectual property rights protection. As a result, the White House announced that preferential tariff treatment under the Generalized System of Preferences program would be withheld for items requested by South Africa until the controversy surrounding the Medicines Act was resolved. The then US Vice-President Al Gore, chair of the US/South Africa Binational Commission, entered the fray, focusing intensely on the issue of intellectual property rights protection. Gore himself was reputedly closely linked to PhRMA and its lobbyists. According to Jamie Love, director of the Consumer Project on Technology, member companies contributed significantly to Gore's Political Action Committee. One of PhRMA's chief lobbyists, Anthony Podesta, was a brother of Clinton's Chief of Staff, John Podesta, a close friend and advisor of Gore. Love also pointed out that Anthony Podesta had worked for David Beier – Gore's chief Domestic Policy Advisor – when Beier was biotech giant Genentech's lobbyist.[16]

Gore's hypocrisy was highlighted in the US press after he stated at a news conference in South Africa that AIDS was a crisis for South Africa that required a 'new level of urgency'. Human rights activists accused him of pretending to be concerned about HIV/AIDS while simultaneously taking actions that would deny people access to essential AIDS medicines.

The US Government consistently threatened to suspend aid to South Africa. The solidly named Omnibus Consolidated and Emergency Supplemental Appropriations Act, 1999, which deals with foreign aid, states: 'Provided further that none of the funds appropriated under this heading may be available for assistance for the central government of the Republic of South Africa, until the Secretary of State reports in writing to the appropriate committees of the Congress on the steps being taken by the US Government to work with the government of the Republic of South Africa to negotiate the repeal, suspension, or termination of section 15C of South Africa's Medicines and Related Substances Controls Amendment Act No 90 of 1997.'[17]

Despite this, and to its credit, the South African Government refused to budge. US consumer activist Ralph Nader accused Al Gore of using bullying tactics to prevent South Africa implementing legal policies designed to expand HIV/AIDS drug access, describing the US administration's attack on the South African law an 'affront to the sovereignty of Third World Nations'.

At the height of the South African pharmaceutical court-case débâcle, Bristol-Myers Squibb announced a gift of $100 million to Harvard and other US universities, UNAIDS, and community projects in South Africa, Botswana, Namibia, Lesotho, and Swaziland. Jamie Love slammed this offer as a 'cynical public relations ploy' pointing out that the gift amounted to less than the $146 million that Bristol-Myers Squibb paid its CEO the previous year.[18]

Protest

The pharmaceutical companies' legal case was weak and civil society resistance was fierce. Under the auspices of the Treatment Action Campaign (TAC), grassroots organizations and the country's largest trade union came together to protest the issue. TAC linked up with international groupings such as ACT UP, Médecins Sans Frontières (Doctors without Borders) and others bringing international pressure to bear. The issue took center stage during the run-up to the 2000 US presidential election campaign during which Gore was repeatedly challenged about it. Its seriousness prompted former Republican supporter Arianna Huffington to remark that: 'Allowing South Africa to license domestic production of the lifesaving drugs, known as compulsory licensing, is one of those rare issues – such as child abuse and drunk-driving – on which there cannot possibly be two sides. After all, the country is suffering from an AIDS epidemic that our own Surgeon-General has compared to "the plague that decimated the population of Europe in the 14th century". The Vice-President's office says it is trying to "help AIDS patients by making sure drug companies maintained profit levels to develop new AIDS medications". But what good are AIDS medications if they can't get to the people with AIDS?'[19]

Recognizing the weakness of its case and the embarrassment of the international attention, the companies backed down. Despite this victory, the South African Government has until recently claimed it cannot afford ARVs, ignoring the options of compulsory and voluntary licensing, parallel imports and generics and thereby angering many AIDS activists. In August 2003, however, the Government finally committed to rolling out a national treatment plan.

Putting the screws on Thailand

One million people in Thailand are HIV-positive. The cost of AIDS treatment in Bangkok costs nearly $700 per month compared with an average monthly wage for an office worker of $110 per month.

Thai law did not allow medicines to be patented until 1994, when the Government was forced to sign the TRIPS agreement as a condition for WTO membership. When Thailand attempted to produce a generic version of the antiretroviral drug ddI, US trade pressure kicked in, threatening sanctions on some of Thailand's key exports such as jewelry and wood unless it used patented medicines. The timing could not have been worse – the Thai economy was reeling in the wake of the Southeast Asian financial crisis. US pressure in 1998 had already stimulated a piece of legislation severely restricting the use of compulsory licenses, way beyond the parameters of TRIPS' minimum standards.[20]

'If Bristol-Myers Squibb, which has not paid for the research and development of the drug, is permitted to maintain its monopoly on ddI and permitted to charge high prices for it, we will be unable to purchase the drug and we will die.' So says the petition submitted by Thai activists to US Health and Human Services Secretary Donna Shalala, calling on her agency to investigate the consumer price for ddI. The drug – a US Government patent – was licensed in Thailand on an exclusive basis to Bristol-Myers Squibb.[21]

NGOs embarked on mass action including demonstrations at the US embassy in Bangkok, demanding the US stop pressuring Thailand to amend its pharmaceutical patent law. The harsh reality was that with 25 per cent of its exports going to the US, the Thai authorities had little choice. They passed special legislation making future compulsory licenses illegal.

India takes on the transnationals

Dr Yusuf Hamied, maverick owner of India's generic drug company Cipla, must surely be Big Pharma's nemesis. In February 2001 he shocked the transnational drug industry by offering to supply a triple cocktail of ARVs for less than $1 a day – a thirtieth of the US patented price. Cipla is now supplying the drugs to a large program treating 10,000 people in Nigeria.

Apparently motivated by witnessing an earthquake that took the lives of 17,000 people in India, Hamied announced that he wanted to do his bit to prevent foreseeable tragedies like AIDS. With a company turnover of $220 million per year and a personal fortune of $550 million, he can clearly afford to be generous, but his offer to sell generics at cut-throat prices has kicked off a price war exposing the gross profiteering of the drug transnationals. GlaxoSmithKline, for example, has threatened to sue Cipla for trying to sell a generic version of its drug Combivir in Ghana. Cipla offered the drug for $1.74 a day. Glaxo cut its price from $16 to $2.

Cipla and other Indian generic manufacturing companies are taking advantage of Indian patent law which protects the *process* by which drugs are made, but not the drugs themselves. If the drugs can be made using a different process from the patented one, the company is covered. Sadly, however, the WTO net is closing and India will have to adopt stronger patent law protection in line with TRIPS and its WTO commitments.

Brazil leads the way

With about 3 million HIV-positive people in the early 1990s, Brazil had the fourth largest number of reported cases in the world. Today, the Brazilian Government has successfully turned back its AIDS epidemic largely because it has defied the transnational drug industry by producing and distributing free ARVs to its PWAs. As a direct result of its aggressive AIDS policy which includes a widespread treatment program, Brazil has managed to reduce the incidence of HIV infection. Since the introduction of ARVs in 1996, the number of hospital admissions due to AIDS-related diseases has dropped by 75 per cent and annual deaths from AIDS have halved. In doing this, Brazil also challenged the prevailing 'global wisdom' that countries of the South do not have the necessary infrastructure to administer ARV medication.

'Brazil can only afford the producing expenditures because we don't pay market prices,' says Health Minister José Serra. 'We put our case to the world and

we've fought for it. And what is our case? It is that
access to medicines is a basic human right.'[22]

According to Dr Paulo Teixeira, director of Brazil's
HIV/AIDS program, 'We started producing these
drugs before the country signed the WTO TRIPS
agreement in 1996. The first consequence was that the
price dropped tremendously – some 80 per cent.'
Teixeira says while the treatment program has cost
Brazil around $300 million of its annual health budg-
et, the program has more than paid for itself by
reducing hospital stays, cutting transmission rates and
enabling thousands to stay in the workforce. The
reduction in the incidence of AIDS-related diseases
has reportedly saved the country $670 million over
three years.[23]

However, the country's action has not gone unchal-
lenged. The US threatened retaliatory measures if
Brazil did not drop its policy on generic drugs and parallel importing. The Bush administration asked for a
WTO disputes hearing, claiming Brazil was in breach
of the TRIPS agreement. Brazil however is well within
its rights having declared AIDS as a national health
emergency. Brazilian law also permits a local company
to manufacture a product, made by a foreign company, if that company fails to initiate production within
Brazil within three years. Predictably, the US filed a
complaint against this law with the WTO. However,
Brazil has won international support for its stance,
including from the UN Human Rights office and the
World Health Organization. The US complaint against
Brazil has subsequently been dropped.

Holding out on life

Big Pharma has also found clever ways to block generic companies from producing cheaper versions of
patented drugs. The transnationals are notorious, for
example, for obtaining new patents on existing drugs
on flimsy pretexts. For example, Bristol-Myers won a
new patent, on anti-anxiety drug Buspar, which did

not even cover the drug itself but rather a chemical compound produced in the body after taking Buspar. It took Mylan (the generic company waiting for approval to sell the cheaper alternative) four months to get a court to invalidate the new patent. In that time, Ron Pollack of Families USA estimates that Bristol-Myers earned another $253 million. A brand company can block the generic competitor from the market for up to two and a half years by filing a patent infringement suit.[24]

Ways forward

Largely in response to bad publicity and the offers by generic manufacturers to slash the costs of HIV/AIDS drugs and supply them to developing countries, pharmaceutical companies have had a run of one-off offers on cheap or free HIV/AIDS drugs to African countries.

In May 2000 five transnationals, supported by WHO and other UN agencies, offered to sell their drugs at greatly reduced prices (although still significantly higher than generics). Many of these offers are yet to bear fruit. Each country is involved in separate negotiations as to how the drugs will be distributed and these have proceeded at snail's pace. But even with an 85 per cent reduction, offered to countries in sub-Saharan Africa by a number of the giants, the costs are still out of reach of most PWAs and their country's health budgets.

Offers to donate provide good PR for drug companies while obscuring other abuses. Providing free drugs for the prevention of mother-to-child transmission, for example, masks excessive prices charged for the same drug as part of HAART. Drug donations and subsidies,

'Access to free medication encourages more people to test themselves and helps curb the spread of the disease.'
Veriano Terto, of Brazilian NGO Associação Brasileira Interdisciplinar de AIDS (ABIA).

reliant on the 'goodwill' of Big Pharma, cannot be seen as a sustainable option.

Ironically, sales to the developing world constitute less than 5 per cent of the industry total and sales to Africa represent just over a paltry 1 per cent. Not only would nothing be lost in providing cheaper drugs or in allowing generic competitors to sell ARVs on a small royalty fee basis, but also the industry could make substantial profits on high volumes of sales. While Big Pharma is concerned that widespread licensing of its products will lead to a global 'black market' in low-priced drugs, perhaps the real fear lies in the fact that consumers in the North will also begin to demand fairer prices. Already US consumer pressure groups are beginning to highlight the gross price disparities.

Activist organizations throughout the world have led aggressive campaigns to force transnationals to cut prices on lifesaving drugs for the poor and to allow for compulsory licensing and parallel imports. This action has brought about a major shift in the world's approach to HIV/AIDS treatment, placing the issue of equity in drug access at the forefront of the international agenda. Activist pressure has already brought about huge price reductions, though not yet low enough for the South to afford. Such pressure has also resulted in international donors, unwilling to fund treatment in the past, now considering doing so. Through the groundbreaking work of these organizations global planning for treatment programs in resource-poor settings is now a reality. UNAIDS and WHO have set a target to expand antiretroviral access to 3 million people by 2005 and together with other multilateral institutions have now set up the International Treatment Access Coalition to assist in reaching this goal.

UNAIDS, in its updated International Guidelines, makes explicit governments' obligations to 'establish concrete national plans on HIV/AIDS related treatment, with resources and timelines that progressively lead to *equal* and *universal* [author's emphasis] access to HIV/AIDS treatment, care and support'. It recognizes that international cooperation and assistance is vital in realizing equitable access to care, treatment and support and calls on governments to contribute towards this end.

In 2001, the UN set up the Global Fund to Fight HIV/AIDS, TB and Malaria in part to assist developing countries access ARV treatment. With an initial target of $10 billion, to be generated through contributions from countries across the globe, in January 2002 the fund stood at just $1.9 billion.

The most just and moral solution would be the wide-scale use of compulsory licensing and parallel importation of cheaper drugs that would loosen the pharmaceutical industry's stranglehold on drug access and ensure that the right to live is not determined by one's pocket. Given the arguments in this chapter, this is also a fair solution. With compulsory licensing, companies would still be paid a royalty fee on sales which would constitute reasonable compensation.

If we do nothing...

Put simply, approximately 40 million HIV-positive people in the world will die if the situation does not change. Life expectancy will continue to drop and countries will be deprived of their most productive people. Millions more children will be orphaned with enormous social consequences. The impact on the economy through the loss of human capital will be accompanied by immense human suffering. Poverty will deepen and the gap between rich and poor will continue to widen.

Prevention, treatment, care and support are a continuum. This is now an internationally recognized fact. Until countries have a treatment program in place, they cannot be said to have a fully comprehensive response to the AIDS epidemic. Until there is equity in treatment access, obituary columns in newspapers in countries of the South will continue to swell with announcements of young people dying in their prime. Treatment has given hope and life to those who can afford it but the battle to moderate the greed of Big Pharma rages on. The final chapter looks to the future and the possibilities for change.

1 Cited in J Achieng, 'Kenya: NGOs seek to import generic drugs from India', *Third World Network,* www.twnside.org.sg/title/generic.htm **2** Personal communication with Dr S Andrews, Johannesburg, 2001. **3** UNAIDS/WHO, *AIDS Epidemic Update,* June 2002. **4** Cited in J Achieng, 'Kenya: NGOs seek to import generic drugs from India', *Third World Network,* www.twn-side.org.sg/title/generic.htm **5** S Sternberg, 'Victims lost in battle over drug patents', *USA Today,* May 24, 1999, cited in P Bond, 'Globalization, Pharmaceutical Pricing and South African Health Policy: Managing Confrontation with US Firms and Politicians' *International Journal of Health Services,* Vol 29, No 4, 1999. **6** J Love, 'Who pays what in drug development', *Nature* Vo 397, No 202, January 21, 1999, cited in P Bond, 'Globalization, Pharmaceutical Pricing and South African Health Policy: Managing Confrontation with US Firms and Politicians' *International Journal of Health Services,* Vol 29, No 4, 1999. **7** D Watson. 'US pharmaceutical companies reap huge profits from AIDS drugs', World Socialist Website, www.wsws.org/articles/1999/jun1999/aids-j05.shtml, 5 June 1999. **8** *Isis News; Special Reports*, No 7/8, February 2001. **9** *The Nation*, 20 August 1999, cited on 'Drug Companies Putting Profits Before Millions of People's Lives', http://www.marxist.com/Africa/aids_drugs_dispute_301.html. **10** S Sternberg, 'Victims lost in battle over drug patents', *USA Today*, 24 May 1999, cited in P Bond, 'Globalization, Pharmaceutical Pricing and South African Health Policy: Managing Confrontation with US Firms and Politicians' *International Journal of Health Services,* Vol 29, No 4, 1999. **11** J Luadano, 'New report links high prescription drug prices to marketing costs, profits and enormous executive compensation', *Families USA Media Center,* www.familiesusa.org/media/press/2001/drugceos.htm **12** G Guenther, 'Federal Taxation of the Drug Industry from 1990 to 1996', Business Taxation and Finance, Congressional Research Service, 13 December 1999 cited in: 'Pharmaceutical Companies Pay Lowest Tax Rate of Any Industry', *The Social Security and Medicare Advisor Newsletter,* April 2000. **13** Médecins Sans Frontières, Health Action International and Consumer Project on Technology. AIDS and Essential Medicines and Compulsory Licensing: Summary of the March 25-27, 1999 Geneva meeting on compulsory licensing of essential medical technologies. Geneva, 9 April 1999, cited in P Bond, 'Globalization, Pharmaceutical Pricing and South African Health Policy: Managing Confrontation with US Firms and Politicians' *International Journal of Health Services,* Vol 29, No 4, 1999. **14** 'Drug Companies putting profits before millions of people's lives', on www.marxist.com/Africa/aids_drugs_dispute_301.html **15** *The Guardian* 12

Feb 2001, on www.marxist.com/Africa/aids_drugs_dispute_301.html **16** P Bond, 'Globalization, Pharmaceutical Pricing and South African Health Policy: Managing Confrontation with US Firms and Politicians' *International Journal of Health Services,* Vol 29, No 4, 1999. **17** Cited in P Bond, op. cit. **18** P Bond, op. cit. **19** A Huffington, 'Pharmacologic AI', on http:/www.ariannaonline.com/columns/files/062899.html. 28 June 1999, cited in P Bond, op cit. **20** Médecins Sans Frontières, Health Action International and Consumer Project on Technology. AIDS and Essential Medicines and Compulsory Licensing: Summary of the March 25-27, 1999 Geneva meeting on compulsory licensing of essential medical technologies. Geneva, April 1999, cited in P Bond, op. cit. **21** 'Thais Protest US Stance on AIDS Drugs', *The Data Lounge*, 6 September 2002, on http:www.datalounge.com/datalounge/news/record.html?record=3474. **22** C Reardon, 'AIDS: How Brazil Turned the Tide', *Ford Foundation Report*, Summer 2002. **23** M Flynn, 'Cocktails and Carnival', *New Internationalist No* 346, June 2002. **24** 'Pushing Drug Profits to the Limit', *CBS News.com*, 26 July 2001, on www.cbsnews.com/stories/2001/07/26/eveningnews/main303607.shtml

5 Turning the tide: responses to the epidemic

'I'm no optimist about the virus. But I simply don't believe, on the basis of personal observation, that we have to face Armageddon. In fact it enrages me the way in which we pile despair upon catastrophe... rendering everyone paralyzed. You don't have to be some pathetic bleeding heart to see the potential strength in these societies at the grass roots, and know that if we could galvanize the governments, indigenous and external, and equip civil society, and address capacity and infrastructure with external resources, then we could defeat this pandemic. It is not beyond our competence.'

Stephen Lewis, UN Special Envoy for HIV/AIDS in Africa.

So far, history will not judge us kindly. Global responses to HIV/AIDS have been criminally apathetic and slow. Millions of lives have been lost while countries have dithered, denying the reality. Yet success stories in parts of the world have demonstrated that the epidemic can be beaten. The steps necessary to do this are now well known. What remains to be done is to 'just do it'.

In 2002, the HIV virus infected 5 million more people. In the same year, 3 million people died of AIDS – more than 8,000 people every day. This would fill over 14 jumbo jets. If these jets were to crash and kill all of their passengers every day for a year, the world would pull out all the stops to end the crisis – no question. After the tragedy of the World Trade Center bombings on 11 September 2001 the West galvanized into action with its 'War on Terror'. Yet more people are dying of AIDS everyday and most of the world acts as if nothing untoward is happening.

Twenty years into the epidemic, it seems clear what needs to be done. Articulating it is the easy part: doing it is obviously harder. But it can be done. Countries such as Brazil, Australia, Thailand, Cambodia, Uganda and the Philippines have reversed their epidemics because they have had the foresight and the political will to do so. But not all these governments responded of their own volition.

Civil society should not be civil

Perhaps the greatest predictor of a nation's response to AIDS is the degree of activism within its civil society. Affecting ordinary people as it does, the pandemic has given birth to social movements that have successfully influenced government policy and implementation on HIV/AIDS. From America to Brazil, Thailand and South Africa, activists have helped propel HIV/AIDS to the top of the news and the international agenda.

While the Brazilian Government is to be commended for providing free antiretroviral (ARV) treatment to its citizens, according to Brazilian AIDS activist Richard Parker: 'If activists had not done all that legal aid and advocacy work in the 1980s and early 1990s, the concept of access to antiretroviral treatment as a basic right of citizenship would be unthinkable.'[1] The Brazilian Government acknowledges as much. In South Africa organizations such as the Treatment Action Campaign took the government to the Constitutional Court to secure the provision of an ARV, Nevirapine, to all pregnant mothers in order to prevent the transmission of HIV from mother to child.

Beyond shaping policy, civil society has also carried the weight of caring for the sick and dying. Noerine Kalleba of UNAIDS lost her husband to the disease and gave up her job as a physiotherapist to fight the epidemic in Uganda. 'We started by setting up a support group (TASO) because we needed to comfort each other. I began to find people with AIDS who had been brought to the hospital and then abandoned there. I thought if AIDS is going to take people's lives but also take people's dignity, as Africans we would have lost more than just life.'[2]

Home-based care programs, where community members are trained to support and look after people who are sick with AIDS, are largely run through the efforts of non-governmental and community-based organizations, many operating on a wing and a prayer. Most rely on volunteers. More resources are needed to help support these vital initiatives. Their provision requires political will and commitment.

Put your money where your mouth is...

The sea-change of the epidemic begins with political will. When it is there, a country can succeed. It mobilizes the resources and provides leadership that can go a long way towards destigmatizing the epidemic – as in Uganda with President Museveni authorizing resources for educational campaigns and speaking about HIV/AIDS in all his public addresses. Decentralized programs reaching villages and open talk on sex and condoms have been the priority, with bold public service advertisements in the mass media and sex education in schools.

We saw in chapter 4 how Brazil took on the powerful transnational drug companies with a decision to provide free ARV treatment for its citizens. By 2000, this commitment had led to a one-third drop in the number of AIDS deaths since the program was introduced in 1996. Former Brazilian president, Fernando Henrique Cardoso set the tone: 'We are not trying to challenge anyone. We don't want to overstep patents [for the antiretroviral drugs provided] at any price. But for the health of our nation, we won't hesitate.'[3]

According to the UNAIDS/WHO 2002 Report, Zambia succeeded in reducing new infections through mass mobilization and awareness campaigns by community and faith-based organizations. In just three years Cambodia made significant inroads into its epidemic in the mid-1990s with infection rates among pregnant women down by almost a third. UNAIDS ascribed this, in part, to a wide condom-use program, as well as steps to counter stigma and reduce people's vulnerability. Unfortunately, lack of information and discrimination still lurk in the minds of many key politicians. Most recently, the deputy minister for the Luapula province in Zambia proposed to round up all HIV-infected people and force them into isolation camps.

No half measures

The ingredients for success are a combination of high-level political commitment coupled with a comprehensive approach to prevention, care and treatment that embraces both community based participation and involvement of PWAs. All components are part of a continuum. Home-based care programs to assist sick people can also bring partners and family in touch with help. It can bring children in distress into contact with a safety net. Treatment programs also have a preventive function by giving an incentive for people to get tested. More people will then know their HIV status and as we have seen, people who know they are HIV-positive are more sexually responsible. This helps prevent more infections. Providing treatment also helps reduce the stigma attached to HIV/AIDS, again helping prevention efforts.

HIV/AIDS is a development issue

While HIV is a virus affecting people's health, it will not be eradicated through a purely medical response. With both socioeconomic roots and impacts, HIV/AIDS has eroded development gains and requires a broad response. The UNAIDS/WHO Report acknowledges that 'addressing the economic, political, social and cultural factors that render individuals and communities vulnerable to HIV/AIDS is crucial to a sustainable and expanded international response'.[4] This includes lofty goals such as halving global poverty, ensuring primary school education for all, and promoting gender equality and the empowerment of women. A total package is vital to success.

When it comes to identifying the problems, everyone is clear on the need to deal with poverty and gender but sadly this understanding does not translate into solutions. Country programs still focus primarily on health, with poverty and more recently gender appearing as footnotes – if at all – on the plan. Yet addressing these issues should take center stage. Without this focus, the impact of other approaches is probably diminished.

Dealing with debt

At a macro level, cancellation of global debt must surely be one of the interventions with the potential to make a vast difference. Debt is crippling sub-Saharan Africa and hitting other poor countries, draining national coffers that should be used in part to confront the burgeoning AIDS epidemic. Neo-liberals are vocal on the potential benefits of globalization yet the reality for most ordinary people is that the rich are getting richer and the poor, poorer. If there are fruits to be gained from globalization, these need to be more equitably distributed. Others would argue for an entirely different world order. At a micro level, targeted anti-poverty programs are needed to generate income and to extend credit and other forms of support to poor communities.

'A woman's place is... everywhere'

As shown earlier, women's low standing places them at greater risk of infection. Gender-based violence and HIV/AIDS sit together like a couple in a bad marriage and are increasingly acknowledged as two mutually reinforcing epidemics (see chapter 2). In their subordinate role, most women cannot insist on safer sex and are therefore particularly vulnerable.

Countries have responded to the crisis in varying

ways; some practical, others potentially damaging. 'Virginity testing' in South Africa is a case in point where girls' genitalia are inspected at public ceremonies and certificates given to those who 'make the grade'. South Africa's Gender Commission calls this 'another form of gender violence', burdening the very people struggling to assert autonomy.

Obviously an HIV vaccine will protect women but remains a long way off. One of the more sensible ideas being explored is the development of vaginally-inserted microbicides – which will kill the virus and can be administered without one's partner's knowledge. Microbicides will give women protection in a world where male partners – arguing they 'won't eat a sweet with its wrapper on' – flatly refuse to use condoms. The bad news is that while microbicides are a good idea, no safe and effective one is yet to be had. With sufficient funds allocated to research, however, they could be available within five years. The female condom is another intervention aimed at giving women more control, although the same constraints would probably apply to its usage as with male condoms because anyone who has ever used one will know that you cannot pretend it isn't there. And of course, women who have been raped should by law have access to antiretroviral treatment.

Gender inequality: the root of the problem

These solutions are important in providing immediate protection for women but they are only 'damage control'. They don't address gender inequality. With this in mind, programs aimed at women's empowerment, human rights education and legislation, gender sensitivity and raising women's self-esteem are growing throughout the world. Early interventions among children and youth to promote equitable and mutually respectful relationships are essential.

Programs for building women's greater autonomy need to go beyond education and gender awareness to broader goals. Geeta Rao Gupta, president of the International Center for Research on Women, explains that: 'Empowerment is information, education, economic opportunities and assets, social support, services, technologies and political participation, all of which help women to take control of their lives...'[5]

Women and girls also have a right to legal protection as a mechanism to help achieve that control. While legislation is obviously not a cure-all, it can help protect women to some extent against a broad range of HIV/AIDS-related discrimination, including violence. The UN's Convention on the Elimination of all forms of Discrimination Against Women (CEDAW) provides a framework for legal reforms and other steps to protect women's human rights. Such reform must apply to both national and traditional and religious law. For example, inheritance laws in some countries allow a deceased husband's family to repossess both the home and his children. In the context of AIDS many women, often infected by their now dead husbands, lose everything. Ugandan activists have managed to secure inheritance rights for widows using CEDAW as an international benchmark. Regretfully, despite almost universal ratification of CEDAW, relatively few countries have incorporated its principles into national legislation.

What about men?

For many, this is the real starting point. Others question the effectiveness of counseling perpetrators of violence against women. However, more projects are engaging men to change behavior and promote respect and equality for women. Many gender activists complain that programs focusing on men divert scarce resources that should be for women. Elizabeth Musaba, a Zambian doctor who has worked for years on violence against women believes this misses the point: 'In Zambia in the 1980s we got nowhere with our family planning program until we began to incorporate men.

We will get nowhere with AIDS if we exclude them. We mustn't lose sight of the ultimate goal which is to build the capacity of women, but we can only succeed if the two aspects are addressed simultaneously.'

McDonald Chapalapata of the Malawi section of Men Against Gender-Based Violence – a network of projects in Namibia, Malawi, Kenya and South Africa – believes their work with men is already bearing fruit. 'Our project brings on board influential men from the judiciary, police, politicians and churches to speak out publicly against gender violence. We have pastors who are preaching respect for women's rights from the pulpit. We run workshops on gender equality and help form village committees which are trained in women's rights and the law. We are definitely starting to see results. In the southern lakeshore district, the village committee arrested a police officer who beat up his mother-in-law and wife. It took great courage to arrest a policeman. As we speak, he is doing time.'

'There's this notion that power is finite,' says Geeta Rao Gupta. 'It's a pie and if you take a piece, then I get less. I like to believe that power is infinite in the long term, so that if you give women power, you are not taking away men's power, you're adding to the power of the entire household, the community, the country.'[6] Perhaps with more projects attempting to shift social norms around gender equality, society will begin to see things more in this way.

While the jury may still be out on whether individual 'perpetrator counseling' works, the HIV/AIDS epidemic will not slow unless everyone takes responsibility, especially men.

Stigma and the defense of human rights

As seen earlier, linking AIDS with sex and death has resulted in an epidemic that is steeped in taboo, silence and stigma. Fear of incurable disease, early associations of the infection with illegal or 'forbidden' practices such as injecting drug use, sex work, multiple sexual partners, homosexuality and sermons on 'divine retribution' have resulted in a stigma which stymies prevention efforts. On the personal front, it makes people feel guilty or ashamed, or scared of the possible discrimination should they be found to be HIV-positive. And this stops them seeking help that could improve their own chances of survival and protect others not yet infected. On the national and international front, stigma stops countries from taking action. Sandra Thurman, head of the White House AIDS Office under President Clinton makes this point: 'This is an epidemic that has been absolutely driven by prejudice. We've been hamstrung in our efforts by racism, by homophobia, by sexism, by class-ism and we have stumbled on every single block; we have not made it over a single obstacle without stumbling.'[7]

One successful strategy to address stigma has been to encourage both high profile and, just as importantly, 'ordinary' people to reveal their HIV status, making HIV/AIDS more visible. Similarly, demonstrations of openness and care from 'role models' help to trash the myths around HIV/AIDS, especially those related to transmission through casual contact. While many saw Princess Diana only as part of the anachronistic British monarchy, a single picture of her embracing a person with AIDS went a long way towards 'normalizing' the epidemic. Some religious leaders are 'breaking the silence' around HIV/AIDS and encouraging openness and compassion amongst their congregations. Another major approach to eradicate stigma focuses on human rights.

HIV/AIDS and human rights

The human rights dimensions of HIV/AIDS are far-reaching. People have the right to be free from discrimination, the right to information, employment, confidentiality and privacy, sexual autonomy, and the right to accessible and affordable medicines to protect the right to life and health (see section on 'Treatment' p 131). All these rights are under threat in various ways in relation to HIV/AIDS. From the early days of the epidemic stories emerged of people being fired or denied work as a result of their HIV-positive status. Incidents of evictions and abandonment were rife. A rash of discriminatory legislation began to appear, restricting international movement of people with HIV or enforcing pre-employment HIV testing.

Pioneers such as Dr Jonathan Mann and Daniel Tarantola of WHO's Global Program on AIDS and Justice Michael Kirby of the Australian Supreme Court were amongst the first to recognize the importance of protecting and promoting human rights in relation to HIV/AIDS. They argued that the epidemic could only be brought under control by breaking the taboos around it and creating a climate of trust whereby people with HIV felt protected. In an enabling environment people would feel more open about testing, disclosing and seeking help. It would break the silence that pushes the epidemic underground, allowing more openness and facilitating easier access to life-saving information and help.

Since those early days, human rights discourse has become integrated into most responses to AIDS with the trend towards discriminatory legislation replaced by laws that explicitly protect these rights. The International Labour Organization (ILO) and WHO developed recommendations to protect the rights of

Telling all in the US

At 62, Barbara has been living with HIV for at least ten years. No one could have been more shocked than she when at age 52 she tested positive for HIV.

Not missing a beat, she told her children, her grandchildren and her great grandchildren. And she told them to get used to it because she was going to speak publicly about it!

Her family has seen tragedy and they have rallied to their mother knowing that AIDS is just another of the struggles that have made her so tough.

http://www.thebody.com/loelpoor/

PWAs in the workplace. The International Guidelines from UNAIDS in 1998 highlighted 12 key areas of HIV-related discrimination and made recommendations to 'assist states in translating international human rights norms into practical observance in the context of HIV/AIDS'. The many human rights instruments such as CEDAW and the Convention on the Rights of the Child are now interpreted within the context of HIV.

Treaties with teeth

Do any of these conventions, treaties and guidelines actually have teeth? Many people say no, but there are clear cases where their presence has made a difference. Countries signing and ratifying them are obliged to bring domestic legislation in line with their principles and there are many instances where these instruments have helped provide a framework for progressive legal judgments.

For example, in Costa Rica a public hospital laboratory refused to undertake testing of people known to be HIV-positive. A group of patients took its case against the hospital to the Constitutional Court which found in their favor and established the right of access to health services for PWAs. Costa Rica has also passed legislation which specifically protects such people against discrimination or degrading treatment. It secures their rights to health and confidentiality and prohibits mandatory tests and discrimination in employment and education. It also provides for condoms to be universally available and stipulates that the Ministry of Health must implement educational campaigns and provide condoms in penitentiaries.

Similarly in South Africa, the Treatment Action Campaign's success in its battle to secure ARV access for the prevention of mother-to-child transmission was won on the grounds that failure to provide such medication constituted a violation of rights as outlined in the South African Constitution, itself heavily influenced by the international human rights agenda.

Unfortunately, some countries have been slow to respond. Section 377 of the Indian Penal Code legislates against homosexuality, sentencing 'whoever voluntarily has carnal intercourse against the order of nature' to up to ten years' imprisonment. Namibia altered a law to nullify a precedent set by a successful legal challenge that forced the Namibian Defence Force (NDF) to recruit a soldier who was refused on the grounds of his positive HIV status.[8]

Despite some successes, legislation is not the whole answer: in many instances a country's civil law may be in conflict with its customary or religious law. This invariably impacts on the standing of women and often on gay rights.

In the light of this, effective reform means dealing simultaneously with civil, customary and religious laws. On top of that, many countries that have signed and ratified the international instruments are still a long way from actually applying them. There is an urgent need to strengthen human rights organizations so that they can push harder for these paper rights to become reality for people affected or infected by HIV/AIDS.

Prevention is better where there is no cure

In the absence of a cure and with no vaccine yet to provide biological protection, it is vital to have programs preventing people from transmitting HIV. Mass communication campaigns, youth education and condom promotion and distribution are some important prevention approaches. As part of a broader response that includes addressing the gender and poverty dimensions of the epidemic, these interventions can make a difference.

> *'I have learned more about love, selflessness and human understanding in this great adventure in the world of AIDS than I ever did in the cut-throat, competitive world in which I spent my life.'*
> **Anthony Perkins, US screen actor, 1932–1992**

Over the years, we have become more sophisticated in our responses. The world is waking up to the fact that frightening campaigns with horror stories of how 'AIDS kills' perpetuate hysteria and drive the epidemic further underground. Wised-up projects have tailored their work to resonate with different groups and needs. Early campaigns in North America targeting gay men with prissy and moralistic messages were replaced by risqué approaches that spoke explicitly of the joys of 'fucking safely'. Advantages of using a condom – like making good sex last longer – replaced the doom and gloom approaches of early campaigns.

Treating sexually transmitted infections (STIs) has proved to be an important mechanism to prevent the transmission of HIV (see chapter 3); voluntary testing and counseling programs which encourage people to be tested for HIV have also been shown to work especially where treatment is available. Various studies have shown that those who receive counseling are more likely to protect themselves by maintaining a healthier lifestyle and seeking early treatment for opportunistic infections if they are HIV-positive. They are also more likely to protect others.

Pre- and post-test counseling provide an opportunity for people to learn about the virus, how it is spread and how it can be prevented. It also helps prepare people for the possibility of a positive test result, one which could change their lives. Information and support relating to the rights of people who are HIV-positive should be integral to this process.

With one third of people with HIV worldwide also infected with tuberculosis, TB is the leading cause of death among people with HIV. The AIDS epidemic is responsible for the global surge in active TB cases and programs aimed at its prevention and treatment are important components of an integrated response to HIV/AIDS. Programs to prevent mother-to-child transmission have also proved highly effective, virtually eliminating pediatric AIDS in many Northern countries. Workplace prevention schemes and outreach to vulnerable groups such as sex workers and truck drivers are also important.

To beat AIDS the world has to put aside its prejudices; there is no place in prevention work for perceived 'moral high ground'. Intravenous drug users, sex-workers and their clients all need and have the right to protection.

Drug-injecting communities and shooting galleries (where users come together to inject) are little paradises for the virus. Brazil, Vietnam, India, Australia and Argentina have achieved a substantial drop in HIV prevalence among such drug users after adopting specific prevention schemes. Gently referred to as 'Harm Reduction Programs' or 'needle exchange programs', they involve swapping free sterile needles for used

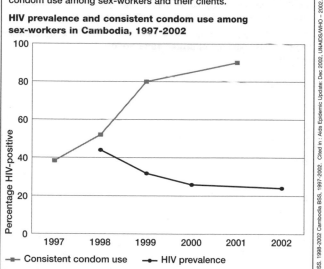

Condom Control

Countries such as Cambodia and Thailand have been able to reverse the upward trend of AIDS through programs promoting consistent condom use among sex-workers and their clients.

HIV prevalence and consistent condom use among sex-workers in Cambodia, 1997-2002

Consistent condom use — HIV prevalence

HSS. 1998-2002 Cambodia BSS, 1997-2002. Cited in : Aids Epidemic Update. Dec 2002, UNAIDS/WHO – 2002.

ones and include counseling, support groups, referrals to drug treatment and medical care. Opponents claim the schemes condone drug use and possession which remain illegal and send the wrong messages to traffickers and potential users. However, research has shown that the programs do not increase drug use. On the contrary, they tend to lead participants to seek help, treatment and other services that generally reduce the habit. Spearheaded by the Netherlands, needle exchange programs now operate in about 40 countries.

Things can change

Where conditions are right and conducive, large-scale behavior change is possible. Perhaps one of the most remarkable examples of this, largely driven by gay

European Centre for the Epidemiological Monitoring of AIDS, HIV/AIDS Surveillance in Europe, 2001. Cited in: 'Young People and HIV/AIDS: Opportunity in Crisis', UNICEF, UNAIDS, WHO, 2002.

Lethal injections

Needles provide a perfect conduit for HIV transmission: rates of infection are soaring in drug-using communities. Research shows that needle exchange programs, which provide injecting-drug users with clean needles, can reduce the rate of HIV transmission.

Reported number of new HIV infections among adolescents (aged 10-19) who inject drugs, 1995-2000

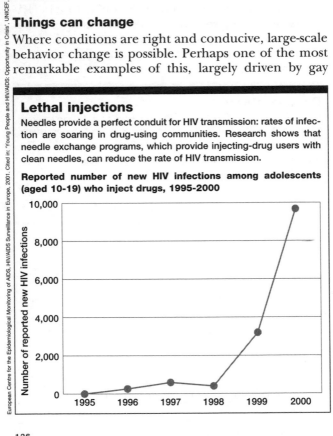

men, took place in San Francisco during the mid-1980s. Huge public awareness drives, closure of the bath-houses (where lots of unsafe sex was happening), and acknowledging the source of people's illness all helped reverse the epidemic in this localized community of gay men.

Around half the monogamous men and about 70 per cent of non-monogamous men reported practicing unprotected anal intercourse in 1983-4. Four years later, those figures dropped to 12 and 27 per cent respectively.[9]

Thailand began to reverse its epidemic trend in only 20 months between 1991 and 1992 by promoting total condom use among sex-workers. Mechai Viravaidya, head of the country's HIV/AIDS Control Program, is famous for his flamboyant awareness-raising initiatives including the establishment of 'Cabbages and Condoms' in Bangkok; the world's only restaurant where you can eat and get condoms simultaneously.

The limitations of 'ABC'

While condoms are the mainstay of most national prevention programs and have helped to curb the epidemic in countries such as Uganda, Thailand and Cambodia, they have their limitations. For a start there are the tricky issues of gender and poverty which either make it impossible or undesirable to insist on condom use if it means losing the man you depend on for your livelihood. It was noted earlier that women who try to get their male partners to use one are accused of being 'prostitutes' or 'sleeping around' and face desertion or violence as a result. Throughout the world, men offer desperately poor sex-workers more money to do it 'flesh to flesh'. The Thai Government's declaration of total condom use for *all* sex workers (brothels that did not comply were shut down) – removed the 'shop around' option for clients. But in the absence of gender equality and in the presence of poverty and rape, the 'ABC' approach to HIV prevention – Abstain; Be faithful; wear a Condom – is just about impossible for many women or girls.

And as we have seen, the fact that children are seen as a person's wealth in many cultures presents another obstacle. Women are under tremendous pressure to be fruitful and multiply, precluding any form of contraception.

In addition, many major religions prohibit the use of contraception. While some religious leaders have used their positions to encourage openness and compassion for PWAs and counsel their congregations in prevention, many refuse to discuss the issue of condoms. However, there are exceptions: in largely Muslim Senegal for example condom use is widely accepted with studies showing high levels of distribution and usage.[10]

Moral maze

Religion and culture can both support and hinder the spread of HIV, as shown in chapter 2. Much of the stigma and blame relates to issues of morality and the perception that a PWA has in some way transgressed both cultural and religious mores. Certain cultural practices, such as female genital mutilation, place women overtly at risk. Their subordinate position also increases their vulnerability. At the same time, culture and religion are also protective. There is some evidence to suggest that male circumcision decreases the transmission of HIV and evidence is emerging of the link between spirituality and positive health behavior[11]. Critically, much of the care and compassion for those who are sick, dying or abandoned through HIV/AIDS comes from faith-based organizations.

Innovative projects have started to revive aspects of traditional culture such as non-penetrative sex encouraged amongst youth in parts of Africa in the past. Some regions have tried to restore the sexuality education that accompanies initiation ceremonies, the rites of passage for many young Africans. Embracing partnerships with traditional and spiritual leaders is essential in the process of reaching out to communities across the globe.

Our children are our future but what future for our children?

Programs focusing on children and youth are important for a number of reasons. Given the power dynamics between adults and younger people in virtually all societies, children are particularly vulnerable to infection through abuse and exploitation. Again, poverty rears its ugly head with many children, mostly girls, entering into unsafe relationships in order to secure their own or their families' survival. Around one million children are forced into the sex trade every year. Rape and child abuse is all too common. These atrocities also call for legislative responses with resources to ensure that laws are implemented.

Also, adolescence is a time of experimentation and risk-taking. Information about one's body, contraception, HIV/AIDS and sex are vital to help young people make informed choices. Such information should be combined with human rights and gender sensitization as part of youth life-skills programs aimed at building the skills and self esteem necessary to assert oneself.

While awareness of HIV/AIDS in general is high, there appears to be a staggering lack of detailed knowledge amongst young people. A study in the Ukraine (see **No room for complacency** graphic p 132) showed that, while 99 per cent of girls had heard of HIV/AIDS, fewer than 10 per cent could correctly identify ways of avoiding sexual transmission. Surveys from 40 countries show that myths abound in over half of all 15-24 year-olds[12], ranging from the belief that HIV is spread by mosquito bites to the frighteningly dangerous misconception that you can tell if someone is HIV-positive by the way they look.

Young people are having sex increasingly early. In many parts of the world large percentages of girls are married before their 18th birthday. Studies of boys aged 15-19 in Brazil, Hungary and Kenya found that over 25 per cent had had sex before they were 15.[13] The younger the age of sexual onset, the greater the likelihood of that sex being unsafe.

Delaying the onset of sexual activity is therefore a priority, and informing young people about it is vital. Contrary to the common belief that this promotes 'promiscuity', experience points to the opposite. It is

Starting young

Children the world over are having sex earlier. Contrary to popular belief, programs which educate young people about sex actually encourage abstinence and less risk-taking behavior.

Percentage of young men and women (aged 15-19) who had sex before age 15, 1998-2001

Measure Demographic and Health Surveys (DHS) 1998–2001; Health Behavior in School-Aged Children Surveys, 1998.
Cited in: 'Young People and HIV/AIDS: Opportunity in Crisis', UNICEF, UNAIDS, WHO, 2002.

both useless and dangerous to our children to bury our collective heads in the sand. Uganda's success in reducing HIV-infection rates has been attributed in large part to open talk about sex. Noerine Kalleba of UNAIDS describes her country's reaction: 'In the early response to the epidemic there was an intense debate whether or not young people should be educated about sex and the prevention of HIV. But I think that debate was a good one to happen early... it led to agreement within families that HIV/AIDS education can be taught at school with the result you find very open sex discussion among young people.'[14]

Measures to protect children include early access to information and programs that develop both the skills and the self-confidence necessary for young people to protect themselves. The promotion of mutually respectful relationships should begin at this early age to help inoculate society against gender discrimination.

Protecting children must also encompass help for young people affected by HIV/AIDS. With the burden of care for sick relatives and siblings often falling on this group, the epidemic is robbing millions of their childhood. Many drop out of school to help with care and are often left destitute after their parents die. Lacking access to health, shelter and food, their lives literally hang in the balance. If unprotected, these kids slip into the margins, vulnerable to abuse, sex trafficking, child labor, drugs and military recruitment. Many land up on the streets. Programs to help them are growing and range from community-based care programs that provide them with practical help to keep them in school, as well as projects that promote a firmer social security safety net.

Health before profits – HIV/AIDS treatment

The degree to which people have access to ARVs and medication to treat opportunistic infections is surely the litmus test of morality in our 21st century world. It is untenable that despite the availability of lifesaving medicine for PWAs, few can afford to buy their lives. Less than 5 per cent of people in need of these drugs in the South are able to get them. This shocking injustice has led to the rise of a new human rights

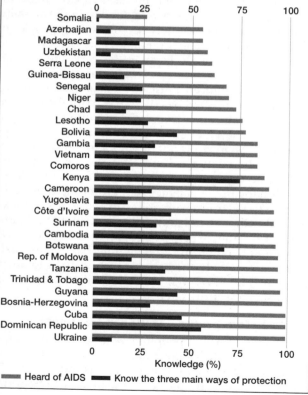

No room for complacency

An alarming number of adolescents do not have the basic information necessary to protect themselves against infection with HIV. However, even with the right knowledge, barriers to protection such as gender inequality and poverty must be addressed.

Percentage of young women aged 15-19 who have heard of AIDS and percentage who know of the three primary ways of avoiding infection, 1999-2001.

Somalia
Azerbaijan
Madagascar
Uzbekistan
Serra Leone
Guinea-Bissau
Senegal
Niger
Chad
Lesotho
Bolivia
Gambia
Vietnam
Comoros
Kenya
Cameroon
Yugoslavia
Côte d'Ivoire
Surinam
Cambodia
Botswana
Rep. of Moldova
Tanzania
Trinidad & Tobago
Guyana
Bosnia-Herzegovina
Cuba
Dominican Republic
Ukraine

Knowledge (%)

▬ Heard of AIDS ▬ Know the three main ways of protection

UNICEF/Multiple Indicator Cluster Surveys (MICS), Measure DHS, 1999-2001. Cited in: 'Young People and HIV/AIDS: Opportunity in Crisis', UNICEF, UNAIDS, WHO, 2002.

movement which focuses on the violation of socio-economic rights related to the HIV/AIDS pandemic, and identifies transnational pharmaceutical companies as major institutional rights violators.[15]

Today, access to drug treatment is viewed not as an optional luxury but rather as a basic necessity in programming in countries both rich and poor. Both UNAIDS and WHO now call for global responses to encompass everything from prevention, home-based and palliative care and the treatment of opportunistic infections to ARV therapy. AIDS treatment is no longer perceived as 'damage control'; its role in prevention is increasingly acknowledged. By providing an incentive for people to be tested, it brings them into contact with support and care that can protect the HIV-positive person as well as others. Although not a cure, by removing the direct association between HIV/AIDS and death, the availability of ARVs reduces fear-related stigma and boosts the success of prevention efforts.

While people can live for many years with HIV through healthy lifestyles and the early treatment of opportunistic infections, there comes a time in the life of every HIV positive person when the only way to stave off the virus is through ARV treatment.

Take HAART

The world is not short of proclaimed 'miracle cures' for HIV/AIDS. Concoctions ranging from industrial chemicals to peach leaves have been punted. Clearly big money is out there to be made. However, as discussed earlier, the only therapy shown conclusively to stem the progression of AIDS is a combination of at least three ARVs or Highly Active Antiretroviral Treatment (HAART).

Since the advent of HAART, epidemics in countries that can afford them have been dramatically altered. Brazil has halved its AIDS-related deaths and cut the number confined to hospital by 80 per cent, since adopting a policy of free ARV provision in 1996. Other countries are following suit. In 2002, Botswana, where 39 per cent of adults are infected, became the first African country to phase in a program of free ARV provision. Senegal, Thailand, Kenya and Zimbabwe are all exploring ways to make the drugs affordable for their people. As seen in previous chapters, this is bringing countries into direct conflict with transnational drug companies and the business interests of wealthier nations. The battle for affordable medication for PWAs has taken center stage in the AIDS arena, highlighting the widening inequality between rich and poor. This is where the real immorality of the epidemic lies – not in the people who have become infected. Other countries that have initiated pilot HAART programs include Côte d'Ivoire, Uganda, Senegal, Zambia, Chile and Vietnam. Many countries in Latin America and the Caribbean have policies or legislation guaranteeing citizens access to ARV therapy. According to the UNAIDS 2002 report Argentina, Costa Rica, Cuba, Uruguay, Honduras and Panama are already providing free and universal access to treatment.[16]

Drug resistance and side-effects are often cited as reasons not to implement large scale ARV treatment programs but as explained in the last two chapters these are not insurmountable obstacles. People on HAART must be monitored for side-effects and switched if necessary to alternative combinations of drugs. Drug resistance is also a problem, but again people can change to a different set of drugs, although eventually they may run out of alternatives. But for most people taking their drugs correctly this only occurs after many years and by that time, new medications are likely to become available.[17] Of great concern is the transmission of resistant strains to other people, thereby limiting their treatment options too.[18]

Delivering the service

A successful HAART program must have trained nurses and counselors, reliable laboratory services and educational programs to support correct drug use. The pharmaceutical industry claims the real barrier to treatment in the South is not the price of drugs but rather the poor state of health systems which it says cannot deliver these services. There is no question that health services in many countries of the South need a complete overhaul – and many have suffered from cuts under structural adjustment programs imposed by the West. However, if we wait until all health services are ready, chances are HAART will not be widely available in our lifetime.

AIDS programs can be used to catalyze infrastructure development with obvious spin-offs for other areas of health and development. This principle has been successfully applied in Brazil for example where many homeless people and those in slum areas have been treated through the creation of small and simple

---

'We are all HIV-positive' – Diamanda Galás

Internationally acclaimed vocalist, pianist, composer and poet, Diamanda was raised in San Diego, California. At the end of the 1970s, she was rolling with a crew of transvestite sex-workers. Calling herself Miss Zina, she received her street education and graduated with honors when she decided that she was a better musician than she was a petty criminal. Diamanda's operatic range and knowledge, combined with her understanding of the outcast, produce a body of art that is both poignant and horrific. 'I think the most important thing is to speak honestly and as well about a situation as I can, and after that, what the audience does with it really is their own business. Because I'm an AIDS activist, I would like to think that what I'm saying could be of inspiration or could be of comfort to people dealing with the epidemic. That's my first thought. As an activist, I have to say my primary goal is connecting to people who are dealing with the epidemic. As far as converting ignorant people, I have to say that I care about it on a political level, I don't care about it on an artistic level.' Her *Masque of the Red Death*, a trilogy of compositions dealing with AIDS, was inspired in part by the loss of her brother and *compadre*, the playwright Phillip-Dmitri Galás. Diamanda's commitment to the struggle against AIDS is tattooed across her knuckles. The ink reads 'We are all HIV-positive,' indicting the world for its complacency.

http://www.diamandagalas.com/press/shout1299.htm

clinics. Without action, creaking health systems will collapse completely from AIDS.

Paul Farmer, co-founder of the Partners in Health (PIH) initiative puts it succinctly: 'The people who say you can't treat the poor with these drugs are just looking for a reason not to do it... the bottom line is that rich countries and governments don't want to pay for poor people. I'm not saying that HIV/AIDS isn't a complex medical disease – it is, but it can be managed with existing medicine and using DOT.'[19] DOT stands for Directly Observed Treatment and is commonly used in the treatment of TB. With the aim of ensuring patients adhere to their treatment regimen, helping the medication to work and preventing resistant strains from developing through non-compliance, PIH has been running a treatment program in Haiti since 1997. It has changed people's lives. Says Teofa, a man on the program, 'There are a lot of people who say: "In such a small, poor country you can't get those drugs, you can't manage them." But for me, it's not true. We are the evidence of the success. There is poverty and we are poor, but that's not a reason to say we can't manage a big thing like this.'[20]

Other programs are demonstrating similar outcomes. Médecins Sans Frontières (MSF) runs a treatment project in Khayelitsha township outside opulent Cape Town. The project has shown that HAART programs can be successfully implemented in poor areas with few resources: there is a five times lower frequency of opportunistic infections in people on medication. 'Look at me. I am black and living in a shack, but I am using the drugs and they are working for me,' said Nontsikelo Zwedala, a 33-year-old mother on the MSF program.[21]

The costs of treating a nation must be weighed up against the costs of not. Beyond the toll of human suffering, these include the impact on an overburdened health system as well as caring for the millions of children who lose their parents to AIDS. There are 14 million such children in the world today, a figure set to double by 2010. The loss of a skilled workforce, a generation of service providers (such as health workers and teachers) and the social impact of a generation of parentless children are almost impossible to measure. Lack of access to ARVs for poor people, while the rich get better, is a clear human rights violation. In recognition of this, and also of the critical role that treatment can play in combating the pandemic, the International Guidelines on HIV/AIDS were updated in 2002 explicitly to include the right of access to affordable ARV treatment. The Guidelines call on governments to 'establish concrete national plans on HIV/AIDS-related treatment, with resources and timelines that progressively lead to equal and universal access to HIV/AIDS treatment, care and support'.[22]

The final analysis

In June 2001, at the UN General Assembly Special Session (UNGASS) on HIV/AIDS, member states committed themselves to a set of targets to halt the epidemic's march. These targets are time-bound: generally, 2003 is the date by which strategies and plans are to be developed; 2005 is the implementation date; and 2010 is the date by which the world should be able to measure impact.

If nothing is done, the world could see in the region of 45 million new infections between 2002 and 2010. But the doomsday predictions are valid only *if we do nothing or don't do enough*. There are millions of people out there trying to make a difference and many of them are. But they cannot sustain their efforts nor make the changes necessary without support.

'*I want my life to be a living testimony that people living with HIV/AIDS can make a difference in life!*'
Sibongile Shabane, co-ordinator of the Siyaphila Support Group for People Living with HIV/AIDS in Pietermaritzburg, South Africa.

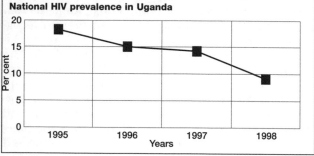

Change is possible

Open dialogue around HIV/AIDS and sex, grassroots mobilization and political commitment at the highest level are some of the factors credited for Uganda's success in reversing its AIDS epidemic.

National HIV prevalence in Uganda

Governments of the North must actively help. But despite grandiose promises at international gatherings to contribute to the Global Fund to Fight HIV/AIDS, TB and Malaria, so far they have not provided enough cash even to make a ripple on the pond.

At the 2002 Conference on HIV/AIDS and 'Next Wave' Countries, the UN's Stephen Lewis made an impassioned plea for what is necessary to turn the tide: 'The truth is that what's literally killing the women and men and children of Africa [and other countries of the South] is the lack of resources... I am strangled by the double standard between developed and developing countries. I am haunted by the monies available for the "war on terrorism", and doubtless to be available for the war on Iraq, but somehow never available for the human imperative... if the Next Wave is to escape the wretched fate of the last wave, then the world and its governments will have to come to their senses.'

1 Quoted in C Reardon, 'AIDS: How Brazil Turned the Tide', *Ford Foundation Report,* Summer 2002. **2** P Brooks, 'An Account of a Catastrophe Foretold', *Steps for the Future* television series, 2001.

3 Quoted in P Rebelo, 'AIDS Drugs: US vs. the World', *Wired News*, 31 May 2001 on http://www.wired.com/news/politics/0,1283, 44175,00.html **4** www.unaids.org **5** Interview with Geeta Rao Gupta by A Kott, 'Gender and the Epidemic', *Ford Foundation Report,* Summer 2002. **6** Interview with Geeta Rao Gupta, op. cit. **7** P Brooks, 'An Account of a Catastrophe Foretold', *Steps for the Future* television series, 2001. **8** M Heywood, 'HIV and AIDS: From the Perspective of Human Rights and Legal Protection', in 'One Step Further – Responses to HIV/AIDS', *Sida Studies* No 7, 2002 **9** McKusick et al, 'Longitudinal Predictions of Reductions in Unprotected Anal Intercourse Among Gay Men in San Francisco: The AIDS Behavioral Research Project.', *American Journal of Public Health,* 80(80), pp.978-83, 1990, cited in A Singhal, E Rogers, 'Combating AIDS Communication Strategies in Action', (Sage Publications 2003). **10** UNAIDS/PennState Project, 'Communications Framework for HIV/AIDS: A New Direction', Geneva, 1999. **11** UNAIDS/PennState Project, op. cit. **12** 'Young People and HIV/AIDS: Opportunity in Crisis' (UNICEF, UNAIDS, WHO, 2002). **13** 'Young People and HIV/AIDS', op. cit. **14** P Brooks, 'An Account of a Catastrophe Foretold', *Steps for the Future* television series, 2001. **15** M Heywood, 'HIV and AIDS: From the Perspective of Human Rights and Legal Protection', in 'One Step Further – Responses to HIV/AIDS', *Sida Studies* No 7, 2002. **16** UNAIDS, 'Report on the Global HIV/AIDS Epidemic 2002' (UNAIDS 2002). **17** 'AIDS: Know the Facts', published by Soul City Institute for Health and Development Communication, The Health Systems Trust, University of Natal 2002. **18** 'AIDS: Know the Facts', op. cit. **19** Anne-Christine d'Adesky. Copyright @ 2001 by the American Foundation for AIDS Research (amfAR) and first displayed on amfAR's Treatment Directory website (www.amfar.org/td) – cited in *New Internationalist* No 346, June 2002. **20** Anne-Christine d'Adesky, op. cit. **21** Quoted in J Lewis's 'A Luta Continua', *Steps for the Future* television series, 2001. **22** www.unaids.org

CONTACTS

INTERNATIONAL

NAM
NAM, Lincoln House
1 Brixton Road
London SW9 6DE, UK
Tel: + 44 20 7840 0050
Fax: + 44 20 7735 5351
Website: www.aidsmap.com

The Global Network of People Living With HIV/AIDS (GNP+)
PO Box 11726
1001 GS, Amsterdam
The Netherlands
Tel: + 31 20 423 4114
Fax: + 31 20 423 4224
Email: infognp@gnpplus.net
Website: www.gnpplus.net

The Global Fund to Fight AIDS, Tuberculosis & Malaria
53 Avenue Louis-Casaï
CH-1216 Geneva-Cointrin
Switzerland
Tel: + 41 22 791 17 00
Fax: + 41 22 791 1701
Email: info@theglobalfund.org
Website: www.globalfundatm.org

The Joint UN Program on HIV/AIDS (UNAIDS)
20 Avenue Appia
CH-1211 Geneva 27
Switzerland
Tel: + 41 22 791 3666
Fax: + 41 22 791 4187
Email: unaids@unaids.org
Website: www.unaids.org

The Global Treatment Access Campaign
Website: www.globaltreatmentaccess.org

Médecins Sans Frontières
Rue de la Tourelle, 39
Brussels
Belgium
Tel: + 32 2 280 1801
Fax: + 32 2 280 0173
Website: www.msf.org

Oxfam
274 Banbury Road,
Oxford OX2 7DZ, UK
Tel: + 44 0870 333 2700
Fax: + 44 1865 312 600
Website: www.oxfam.org.uk

Panos Institute
9 White Lion Street
London N1 9PD,UK
Tel: + 44 0 20 7278 1111
Fax: + 44 0 20 7278 0345
Email: info@panoslondon.org.uk
Website: www.panos.org.uk

International HIV/AIDS Alliance
Queensberry House
104-106 Queens Road
Brighton BN1 3XF, UK
Tel: + 44 1273 718 900
Fax: + 44 1273 718 901
Email: mail@aidsalliance.org
Website: www.aidsalliance.org

Action for Southern Africa (ACTSA)
28 Penton Street,
London, N1 9SA, UK
Tel: + 44 20 7833 3133
Fax: + 44 20 7837 3001
Email: actsa@actsa.org
Website: www.actsa.org

AFRICA

SAFAIDS
17 Beveridge Road,
Avondale
Harare, Zimbabwe
Tel: + 263 4 336193/4
Fax: + 263 4 336195
Website: www.safaids.org.zw

Journalists Against AIDS (JAAIDS) Nigeria
1st Floor, 42 Ijaye Road,
Ogba, Lagos, Nigeria
Tel: + 234 1 7731457
Fax: + 234 1 4921292
Website: www.nigeria-aids.org

Treatment Action Campaign
34 Main Road
Muizenberg 7764
South Africa
Tel: + 27 21 7883507
Fax: + 27 21 7883726
Email: info@tac.org.za
Website: www.tac.org.za

The AIDS Support Organization (TASO)
PO Box 10443
Kampala, Uganda
Tel: 256 41 567637
Fax: 256 41 566704
Email: tasodata@imul.com
Website: www.taso.co.ug

AOTEAROA/NEW ZEALAND

Oxfam
Level 1, 62 Aitken Terrace,
Kingsland, Auckland
Tel: + 64 9 355 6500
Fax: + 64 9 355 6505
Website: www.oxfam.org.nz

New Zealand AIDS Foundation
Website: www.nzaf.org.nz

AUSTRALIA
Oxfam Community Aid Abroad
1st Floor, 156 George Street
Fitzroy, Melbourne
Victoria 3065
Tel: + 61 3 9289 9444
Fax: + 01 0 0419 5318
Email: enquiries@caa.org.au
Website: www.caa.org.au
Australian Federation of AIDS Organizations (AFAO)
Level 1, 222 King Street,
Newtown, NSW 2042
Tel: + 61 2 9557 9399
Fax: + 61 2 9557 9867
Email: afao@rainbow.net.au
Website: www.afao.org.au

CANADA
Canadian AIDS Society
309 Cooper St. 4th floor
Ottawa, ON K2P 0G5
Tel: + 1 613 230 3580
Fax: + 1 613 563 4998
Email: casinfo@cdnaids.ca
Website: www.cdnaids.ca
Canadian HIV/AIDS Legal Network
417 Saint-Pierre Street, Suite 408
Montréal, Québec H2Y 2M4
Website: www.aidslaw.ca

LATIN AMERICA
Grupo Pela Vidda
Av. Rio Branco, 135
Grupos 709/713 - Centro, 20.090-002
Rio de Janeiro, Brazil
Tel: + 55 21 518 3993
Fax: + 55 21 518 1997
Website: www.pelavidda.org.br
Associação Brasileira Interdisciplinar de AIDS (ABIA)
Tel: + 55 21 2223 10 40
Fax: + 55 21 2253 84 95
Website: www.abiaids.org.br

The Agua Buena Human Rights Association
PO Box 366-2200
Coronado
Costa Rica
Tel: + 506 234 24 11
Website: www.aguabuena.org
The Huesped Foundation
Angel Peluffo 3932,
Buenos Aires, Argentina
Tel: + 54 11 4981 7777
Fax: + 54 11 4981 7777
Email: fhuesped@huesped.org.ar
Website: www.huesped.org.ar
REDLA
Calle 8 No. 22-60
Cali, Colombia
Tel: + 57 2 5142211
Fax: + 57 2 5142208
Email: info@redla.org
Website: www.redla.org

UK
See under 'International'

US
San Francisco AIDS Foundation
995 Market St, #200
San Francisco, CA 94103
Email: feedback@sfaf.org
Website: www.sfaf.org
ACT UP (AIDS Coalition to Unleash Power)
332 Bleecker St, Suite G5
New York, NY 10014
Email: actupny@panix.com
Website: www.actupny.org
Health GAP (Global Access Project)
511 E.5th St, #4
NYC, NY 10009
Tel: + 1 212 674 9598
Fax: + 1 212 208 4533
Email: info@healthgap.org
Website:www.healthgap.org

BIBLIOGRAPHY

Paul Farmer, *Infections and Inequalities: the Modern Plagues* (University of California Press 1999).

Tony Barnett and Alan Whiteside, *AIDS in the Twenty-First Century: Disease and Globalization* (Palgrave Macmillan 2002).

Jonathan M Mann and Daniel JM Tarantola Eds, *AIDS in the World II: Global Dimensions, Social Roots, and Responses* (Global AIDS Policy Coalition, Oxford University Press 1996).

AIDS and Men: taking risks or taking responsibility? (Panos Institute and Zed Books 1998).

Susan Sontag, *Illness as Metaphor and AIDS and Its Metaphors* (Anchor Books/Doubleday 1990).

Laurie Garrett, *The Coming Plague: Newly Emerging Diseases in a World out of Balance* (Penguin Books 1995).

Index

Index

Index